The Influence of Aural Training in Music on the Perceptive Performance of Adult Learners' Sound-Discrimination Abilities in an Unknown Foreign Language

European University Studies
Europäische Hochschulschriften
Publications Universitaires Européennes

Series XXI
Linguistics

Reihe XXI Série XXI
Linguistik
Linguistique

Vol./Bd. 369

PETER LANG
Frankfurt am Main · Berlin · Bern · Bruxelles · New York · Oxford · Wien

Friederike Flottmann

The Influence of Aural Training in Music on the Perceptive Performance of Adult Learners' Sound-Discrimination Abilities in an Unknown Foreign Language

PETER LANG
Internationaler Verlag der Wissenschaften

Bibliographic Information published by the Deutsche Nationalbibliothek
The Deutsche Nationalbibliothek lists this publication in the Deutsche Nationalbibliografie; detailed bibliographic data is available in the internet at http://dnb.d-nb.de.

Zugl.: Dortmund, Techn. Univ., Diss., 2010

D 290
ISSN 0721-3352
ISBN 978-3-631-61353-5

www.peterlang.de

to
my family

Preface

The present book is the result of a project which seems to have grown bigger by the course of its progression. This project would not have been manageable without the support, the encouragement and the advice from experts, family, friends and volunteers who consented to taking the time and effort to be the subjects of the study. I am deeply thankful to everyone who helped making this project work.

First and foremost, Prof. Dr. Jürgen Kramer, the supervisor of my dissertation project, was always available with advice and answers and besides showing great patience, he was always sincerely interested in my project. Furthermore, Prof. Dr. Günther Rötter and JProf. Dr. Uwe Ligges were very helpful when taking time to answer my questions on the musical side of the project and on the statistical evaluation. Dr. Henning Sternemann took a lot of time and effort in programming the computer program ToSCA, which was used as the interventive step in the course of the study. Volkmar Frinken took charge of programming the web-environments for the online sound-discrimination tests, which were used as pre- and post interventive instruments of measurement. Heli Duer, as a native speaker of Finnish, helped out in answering questions on the Finnish language, which was used as the test language, and volunteered to be recorded to appear as the voice of the sound-discrimination tests. Uwe Geitner made his studio available for the recording of the Finnish words and phrases. Many friends and friends' friends helped finding suitable subjects for the study, took part in the study, helped testing the beta version of ToSCA or helped proofreading. And finally, I am cordially thankful for all the patience, support and encouragement I received from my family, my boyfriend, my friends and other PhD students at the PhD network of the culture-studies faculty at Technische Universität Dortmund.

Dortmund, September 2010

Friederike Flottmann

Table of Contents

Index of Figures

Index of Tables

Index of Abbreviations

bpm	beats per minute
BLDT	Bremer Lautdiskriminationstest
cat	category
CPH	Critical Period Hypothesis
ci	confidence interval
dB	decibel
diff	difference
FL	foreign language
gd	grade of difficulty
H-LAD	Heidelberger Lautdifferenzierungstest
ibid.	ibidem
incr	increase
LUT	Lautunterscheidungstest
qac	questions answered correctly
SL	Second Language
SSPDT	Speech Sound Pattern Discrimination Test
ToSCA	Training of Sound Contrasting Abilities

1 Introduction

The present study shall investigate in how far human perceptive abilities in foreign languages can be enhanced by non-theory based aural training in music. It is hypothesised that a music intervention of the type described below can improve human sound-discrimination abilities, which are essential for the comprehension of names, words and expressions in an unknown foreign language.

In contrast to other concepts involving music in foreign-language learning such as the suggestopedic / suggestological approach[1], in which music is applied for memory-training purposes, the *Mozart-Effect* theory[2], which employs music to enhance concentration abilities, or pedagogical concepts as described by Cranmer and Laroy[3] involving music for motivational purposes, this study aims to determine the hearing-sensitisation effect of aural training in music. The hypothesis suggests that the aural perception of a spoken foreign language can be enhanced by musical hearing training aimed at the improvement of the subjects' sound-discrimination abilities in pitch, tempo, rhythm, melody and harmony.

This study specifically aims to examine the performance of adult learners, i.e. learners far beyond the critical age window for language learning as described by Singleton and Ryan[4], Moyer[5] and many other authors. Even though large parts of the critical age theory refer to the active side of language learning, namely pronunciation abilities and potential native-like performance in a foreign language which is acquired at an early stage in childhood, according to most authors, before the age of 12, it is interesting to examine to what extent it is possible to train the sound-discrimination abilities of learners well beyond the critical age and to sensitise them to the sounds of a language previously completely unknown to them.

As described by Koelsch et al.[6], musical information is, to a large extent, processed in the brain areas also involved in, and previously believed to be exclusive networks for, language processing in the human brain. A musical hearing training of the type described below aims at specific training of the brain areas in question and thus seems to promise beneficial effects on language processing in the brain. It has been shown that musical syntax, i.e. the melodic and harmonic context in which tones and chords appear, is processed in Broca's area, which was originally known to be one of the brain areas for linguistic syntactic processing.[7] Furthermore, Douglas and Willats were able to provide evidence for a positive effect of rhythmic training on literacy skills for both primary-school children and adults.[8] In light of these studies, it is interesting to examine whether and to what extent one-sided, i.e. musical, training of the brain areas related to both music and language processing can influence the aural perception of language and in particular the discrimination between and the

1 cf. e.g. Bancrof, W. Jane (1999) and Brislan, Patrick S. (1990)
2 cf. e.g. Campbell, Don G. (2001)
3 Cranmer, David; Laroy, C. (1992)
4 Singleton, David; Ryan, L. (2004)
5 Moyer, Alene (2004)
6 Koelsch, Stefan et al. (2002)
7 cf. Maess, Burkhard et al. (2001)
8 cf. Douglas, Sheila; Willats, P. (1994)

recognition of previously unheard and thus entirely unknown sound patterns in a foreign language.

Sound-discrimination ability constitutes only one factor of language perception and language learning. This factor, however, is essential for the acquisition of a new language with previously unknown sounds and sound combinations. Only the ability to distinguish between perceived speech sounds and to recognize them in different contexts will enable the language learner to eventually understand utterances in the foreign language. Sound-discrimination abilities do not only comprise the differentiation between and the recognition of different vowels or consonants or voiced and voiceless versions of consonants, such as [t] in contrast to [d], but often also differences in tempo for single or double consonants or vowels and even differences in intonation. The Chinese language, e.g., makes use of four different kinds of intonation: an even tone, a rising tone, a falling tone and a bent first rising then falling tone, while differently intonated syllables carry completely different meanings. For example, the syllable *yi* means *one*, if pronounced with an even intonation, *to move*, if pronounced with a rising intonation, *chair*, if pronounced with a bent intonation and *one hundred million*, if pronounced with a falling intonation.[9] The extreme difference in meaning between one and one hundred million differentiated by what otherwise may be looked at as "only" the intonation of the syllable is obvious. In Finnish, the language applied in the context of this study, the differentiation between double and single vowels and consonants plays an important role. For example the words *tili*, *tiili* and *tilli* have entirely different meanings: *bank account*, *brick* and *dill*.

Methods for testing and training of music and speech perception are numerous and versatile. Musicality tests as well as aural training concepts in music have a long history and have experienced considerable development over the years, a fact especially true for aural training programs in music ranging from teacher-centred approaches in a classroom situation to free online training programs for self-study application. However, the very special requirements in the context of this study necessitated the development and application of a new kind of aural training program as well as a new testing method for sound-discrimination abilities suitable for the training and testing of novices in both music education and the tested language.

In the course of the present study, 50 subjects, students of non-linguistic degree programmes and without any prior instrumental or vocal training, took part in two sound-discrimination tests at an interval of two weeks, with 25 subjects taking part in a two-week aural training program in music between the two tests. All subjects took part in a survey on their linguistic education and their musical habits prior to the examination as well as in a survey on their estimated performances in both sound-discrimination tests after the examination. It was expected that all subjects would show better performance in the second test due to familiarisation with the new language. The trained group was expected to improve more than the control group based on their musical sound-discrimination training. Furthermore, it was expected that subjects with a broadened taste of music styles would be more receptive to the aural training intervention. Subjects of the trained group were expected to be more likely to estimate their performance in the second test as

9 example from Peiyuan, Li; Yuan R. (1979)

improved as opposed to their performance in the first test than subjects of the control group.

In the following, a brief outline on previous observations of similarities between the two domains of language and music will be given followed by a placement of sound-discrimination abilities' role in the context of speech perception and language learning. Subsequently, an overview of previously applied and the here introduced sound-discrimination test methods will be presented as well as different concepts and methods of aural training in music including the training program designed for the present study. The structure, hypotheses and results of the study will be discussed in depth in the second half of the thesis.

2 Music and Language – Their Interconnectivity from the Neuroscientific, the Developmental Psychological and the Pedagogical Points of View

The similarities and the interconnectivity between music and language, the two acoustic means of conveying meaning, are moving into the focus of attention in many fields of research beyond the domains of education and developmental psychology hitherto chiefly involved in the discussion about the use of one for the benefit of the other. The increasing interest in the beneficial potential of music practice and listening on both productive and receptive aspects of language application and acquisition has been triggered by recent discoveries in neuroscience providing evidence for cerebral activity during music processing[10] in brain areas earlier believed to exclusively process language.[11] Previous to these recent neuroscientific findings, the effects of memorising and concentrating were the main focus of research in context with non-musical outcomes of music instruction and practice. To Sundberg "These [newly found] similarities are not unexpected." He argues that "[s]peech and music are the two main forms of organized interhuman communication by means of acoustic signals. The mind arranging these signals and the mechanism perceiving them is the same in both."[12]

Parallels between music and speech have not been discussed without considering the differences between these two forms of acoustic communication. Since the centre of interest of the present study lies in the similarities between music and language, only a few of these distinctions shall be summarised at this point. The role of semantics is by far not as clearly defined in music as it is in language. Sundberg notes that there is no one-to-one relation between musical phrases and their meanings as there is in language, leading him to the conclusion that "vocabulary seems limited in music"[13] and "the semantics of music seems both fragmentary and optional. The essence of music lies beyond such meanings. This is quite unlike language, where the meaning is normally quite essential"[14]. Sundberg also sees a difference between music and language in the role of structure: "[i]n language, structure serves the purpose of conveying the linguistic message. In music, structure is a goal of its own."[15] Structure, or more precisely grammar, has been an issue for Baroni as well, who concluded his comparison between musical and linguistic grammars by distinguishing musical grammars from linguistic grammars in the way that "[o]ne of their main properties (one which strongly distinguishes them from linguistic grammars) is their high level of mobility, their

10 For further information on the processing of music in the brain, refer to e.g. Cross et al. (1985), Griffith (2003), Krumhansl and Toiviainen (2003), Lee (1985), Parsons (2003), Samson and Ehrlé (2003), Tervaniemi (2003), Tillmann et al. (2003), Watkins and Dyson (1985) and Williams (1981).

11 For detailed explanations on auditory processing in the brain, refer to e.g. Bharucha (1991) and Bellis, Teri J. (1997).

12 Sundberg (1990)

13 ibid.

14 ibid.

15 ibid.

continuous disposition to modify their rules."[16] In the context of human survival, the roles of music and language could not be more different according to Brown, who summarises them by stating that "minimal linguistic skills [...] are essential to survival. Minimal musical skills are not essential"[17]. In the sense of the communicative role of music and language, Brown states rather globally and probably with the average human for whom musical skills are not essential in mind that "[l]anguage is not specific to one sense modality in the way that music is" [18]. The role of pitch in the processing of music and language is one of the aspects investigated by Patel and Peretz, who summarised the different roles with regard to pitch by stating that "musical pitches are used to make melodies, in which the relations between pitches over extended sequences is of central importance. Linguistic tones, in contrast, act as localised semantic and grammatical signals"[19]. In terms of brain processes, the authors finally conclude that "the processing of tonality appears to draw on resources used uniquely by music."[20]

In the context of various studies on differing aspects of the interconnectivity between music and language, one of the main problems hitherto not satisfactorily solved is the attempt to link specific subcategories of language to designated aspects of music. While a one-to-one assignation of extremely detailed, single aspects of one domain to aspects of the other is not very likely, global distinctions have been found for the assimilated processing of all timing-related aspects of music, i.e. rhythm, metre, tempo, etc., and the mastery of literacy on the one hand and all space-related aspects of music, i.e. pitch, melody, harmony, etc., and phonemic, semantic and syntactic processing on the other hand. Although other attempts to find parallels to linguistic phenomena such as grammar, syntax, semantics, etc. in music have also been made, they must be considered with caution. Parallels, though they might be drawn, should remain within the specific limits of a musical piece's historical and cultural background and probably even within the limits of compositional styles and single composers comparable to different languages, developmental states of languages and literary styles. Baroni sums up this problem by reasoning that "musical grammar is not an absolute concept: it is a set of rules, valid for a particular group of users"[21].

Previous studies have investigated both the receptive strategy of music application for potential benefits in the language domain and the productive strategy of active participation in the music. However, a central point of interest in many studies, regardless of the approach, has been the development of listening skills. "The development of good listening skills is basic to language learning"[22] as Birkenshaw concisely phrases one of the main purposes underlying the motivation for many studies including this one.

16 Baroni (1990)
17 Brown (1981)
18 ibid.
19 Patel and Peretz (1997)
20 ibid.
21 Baroni (1990)
22 Birkenshaw (1990)

2.1 Rhythm, Timing, Tempo and Literacy

The question of similarities and commonly shared strategies in the processing of the time-related aspects of music and literacy has been at the centre of interest especially in the context of reading difficulties in children learning to read their mother tongue. Comparatively few studies have ventured further to examine potentially shared processes of literacy in foreign languages and rhythmic abilities. However, "the temporal and accentual patterning of sound"[23], a definition of rhythm issued by Patel and Peretz, seems a rather central aspect in the mastery of a foreign language.

The application of rhythm-focused music instruction has been investigated in the context of its role as a treatment for dyslexic children and as a general method for the enhancement of children's reading abilities.[24] While McCarthy generally advises the inclusion of musical elements in language education in his teaching conception underlining the beneficial effect of music on "word recognition, comprehension, reading study skills, and literary comprehension"[25] and Douglas and Willats were able to confirm an "association between rhythmic ability and reading"[26] in their study carried out on seven- and eight-year-old children, leading them to the conclusion that "training in musical skills is a valuable additional strategy for assisting children with reading difficulties"[27], Overy et al. compared "different types of musical timing skills amongst dyslexic children and control children, in order to identify whether there is a particular area in which music remediation work should concentrate."[28] When testing the subjects' rhythm, metre, rapid and pitch skills, the authors discovered that "rapid timing skills and rhythm skills are areas of particular difficulty for dyslexic children"[29].

Gromko, on the other hand, focused on the aspect of phonemic awareness in the context of children's reading abilities and investigated the effect of instruction in music additional to the children's regular reading instruction based on her assumption that "[p]honemic awareness [...] may be the mechanism that explains the relationship of music instruction to reading skill."[30] Gromko, however, did not exclude the rhythmic factor from her hypothesis: "[w]hen children learn to discriminate fine differences between tonal and rhythmic patterns [...], they will benefit [...] in skills related to the processing of sound shown to be necessary for reading."[31] After the testing of several aspects involved in phonemic awareness, here defined as "the ability to recognize that a spoken word consists of individual sounds

23 Patel and Peretz (1997)
24 For examples of pedagogic conceptions integrating music in the teaching of other subjects, refer to e.g. Birkenshaw (1990), Cranmer and Laroy (1992), Goldberg and Scott-Kassner (2002), Pallasmaa (1990) and Whitaker (1994).
25 McCarthy (1985)
26 Douglas and Willats (1994)
27 ibid. (1994)
28 Overy et al. (2003)
29 ibid.
30 Gromko (2005)
31 ibid.

or phonemes"[32], Gromko was able to show a "significant gain [...] for phoneme-segmentation fluency", the ability to split up heard words into their phonemes.

Investigations on cognitive strategies for the mastery of perception have been carried out e.g. by Repp[33] and Saffran et al.[34] comparing listening strategies of language perception with strategies of music perception. Repp constitutes the general receptive process, whether concerning music or speech, as a sequence of the events of perception, partition, organisation and interpretation wherein the organisation of incoming sounds happens by either integration or segregation, which occurs on the basis of the listener's receptive experience. Repp eventually distinguishes between two major listening approaches: phonetically analytic listening and listening for the acoustic input's meaning and message. In the case of music, this division of listening approaches leaves the question of how to understand the musical message, leading Repp to the conclusion that "[i]f it [the musical message] is taken to be the sound structure per se, then the most analytical listener will receive the most information. However, if the message is taken to be the emotional content, then the synthetic, unreflecting listening may yield maximum returns."[35] Saffran et al. went more into detail and carried out a very specific investigation into cognitive strategies in perceptive processing. In pursuing the question "whether a learning mechanism which contributes to the acquisition of one aspect of language, word segmentation, can also subserve learning in another domain, the grouping and segmentation of tonal sequences"[36], the authors were able to demonstrate that "adult learners readily group sequences of auditory events in the same manner, regardless of whether the input is linguistic (syllables) or non-linguistic (tones)."[37] This phenomenon was attributed to the strategy of expectancies and probabilities, i.e. anticipating potential acoustic events after the perception of certain acoustic information in terms of likelihood of occurrence or, as the authors phrase it, "a mechanism computing [...] probabilistic information is implicated in this segmentation process."[38] The same domain-independent effect could also be shown for children and thus the authors were able to provide "striking evidence for the similarity of statistical learning in segmenting tone sequences and syllable sequences"[39], which lead them to the conclusion that "at least part of the machinery involved in natural language learning may be shared with other pattern learning processes."[40]

32 Gromko (2005)
33 Repp (1990)
34 Saffran et al. (1999)
35 Repp (1990)
36 Saffran et al. (1999)
37 ibid.
38 ibid.
39 ibid.
40 ibid.

2.2 Melody, Harmony, Pitch and Syntactic / Semantic Processing

The processing of the space-related aspects of music has been shown to bear parallels with the processing of the larger sense units in speech responsible for meaning and structure. In this sense, e.g. melody processing has been compared with syntax processing, melody production with sentence production and melodic abilities have been analysed in context with the ability to use prosodic information as a means of understanding foreign languages in particular and of processing linguistic intonation in general.[41] When investigating harmonic processing, parallels to the processing of language, especially to the processing of syntactic information, have been shown.[42] The processing of pitch-related information has been of interest in comparisons with phonetic processing and with linguistic intonation.[43] Furthermore, music has been applied to test its ability to activate semantic-representation areas in the brain.[44] And finally, training in music has been of large interest in the context of memory enhancement, especially in the context of the suggestopedic approach to foreign-language learning for the benefit of enhancing verbal memory and verbal learning.[45]

Melodic processing and melodic production have been shown to share activity in identical, homotopic or adjacent brain areas with syntactic processing and syntactic production respectively and melodic abilities were also found to correlate with linguistic intonation abilities. In an attempt to find an explanation for the apparent contradiction in the question of parallels between linguistic syntactic processing and musical syntactic processing between data collected in neuropsychological studies and in studies using neuroimaging, Patel was able to show an overlap in the brain areas involved in the processing of syntactic information, i.e. an overlap in operations conducted on the base of knowledge forming new synapses, but not for the representation of syntax in the brain, i.e. long-term structural knowledge based on already present synaptic connections, syntax here being defined as "a set of principles governing the combination of discrete structural elements (such as words or musical tones) into sequences"[46]. Parallels between the productive side of speech and music processing have been investigated in a study by Brown, Martinez and Parsons in which amateur musicians were asked to improvise melodies and sentences in response to acoustically presented melodies and sentences.[47] The authors were able to show "activations in nearly identical functional brain areas"[48] for the production of melodies and sentences, with the main differences between the two domains consisting of lateralisation tendencies, which, however, were shifted with different degrees of

41 cf. Patel and Peretz (1997), Becker (1999), Patel (2003), Brown et al. (2006)
42 cf. Koelsch et al. (2002), Maess et al. (2001)
43 cf. Patel and Peretz (1997), Zatorre et al. (1992)
44 cf. Koelsch et al. (2004)
45 cf. Ho et al. (2003), Brislan (1990), Chan et al. (1998)
46 Patel (2003)
47 cf. Brown, Martinez and Parsons (2006)
48 ibid.

musical expertise.[49] In sum, the authors conclude that "not only do music tasks activate right hemispheric areas homotopic to classic left hemispheric language areas [...] but many music tasks elicit bilateral activations that appear to border on or coincide with left-hemispheric – presumably language-specific – areas"[50]. In examining the apparent connection between pupils' musical abilities and their foreign-language learning success, Becker was able to show a correlation between pupils' musical melodic abilities and their ability to make use of prosodic information in foreign-language sentences, reasoning that the connection between their musical and linguistic abilities lies in the use of prosodic information, which indicates a shared neuropsychological process in dealing with melodies and prosodic linguistic information.[51] These findings are in accordance with a comparison of melodic contour, i.e. "the general shape of melodic line [...] without regard to exact pitch intervals"[52], and linguistic intonation carried out by Patel and Peretz, who were able to show "an association between performance on musical contour and linguistic intonation tasks, arguing for some common neural contribution to both types of task."[53]

Linguistic syntactic processing has also been compared with the processing of harmonic progressions in music, especially in the context of unexpected events in an otherwise musically logical cadence. Maess et al. attempted to localise "the neural substrates that process music-syntactic incongruities"[54] by inserting dissonant, out-of-key chords in the process of an otherwise harmonic cadence and were able to show activity in Broca's area and its homologue in the right hemisphere, previously known as the brain areas for the processing of linguistic syntactic input. Thus the authors concluded "that complex rule-based information is processed in these areas"[55] rather than only linguistic information. Koelsch et al. ventured further in the field of processing unexpected events in a harmonic cadence by dividing the disturbance factors into different categories, i.e. dissonant clusters, gradual modulation to a different key and sudden change of instrumentation.[56] For the processing of music in the brain, the authors were able to show an involvement of the right superior temporal gyrus responsible for the processing of pitch, the posterior superior temporal gyrus responsible for the perception of pitch, the anterior superior temporal gyrus responsible for the processing and representation of melody, the right frontal operculum representing the working memory for pitch and the left hemispheric brain areas responsible for the processing of sequential sounds, stressing that "[t]he interdependence of the structures activated in the present study has so far only been observed for the processing of language."[57] As a conclusion of these shared brain networks, which were also able to be shown for non-musicians,

49 For further information on brain changes due to musical practice and expertise, refer to e.g. Gruhn and Rauscher (2002), Pantev et al. (2003), Pascual-Leone (2003), Peretz (2003), Rauschecker (2003), Schlaug et al. (1995), Schlaug (2003), Stewart et al. (2003), Stewart et al. (2004) and Strickland (2002).

50 Brown et al. (2006)

51 cf. Becker (1999)

52 Patel and Peretz (1997)

53 ibid.

54 Maess et al. (2001)

55 ibid.

56 cf. Koelsch et al. (2002)

57 ibid.

the authors suggest that "since the same neuronal network processes musical and linguistic information, the human musical experiences might implicitly train the language network."[58]

Although certainly not independent from harmonic and melodic progression, pitch, as an isolated phenomenon, has been in the centre of interest in comparisons with linguistic pitch, i.e. intonation, as already introduced above, and with phonetic processing. The roles of pitch in music and language are different, as pointed out by Patel and Peretz: "musical pitches are used to make melodies, in which the relations between pitches over extended sequences is of central importance. Linguistic tones, in contrast, act as localised semantic and grammatical signals"[59]. While supporting previous findings revealing the left-hemispheric activity in the processing of both musical and linguistic pitch, the authors suggest that due to the two different functions "these two forms of pitch may be processed separately within the left hemisphere"[60]. Finally, Patel and Peretz conclude that "the processing of pitch contour employs some of the same neural resources in music and language"[61] with the important restriction that "the processing of tonality appears to draw on resources used uniquely by music"[62]. Zatorre et al. were able to show different processing stages for acoustic information reaching the brain in an examination of the perceptive processing of different aspects of one and the same speech signal.[63] They were able to show that "auditory information undergoes discrete processing stages, each of which depends on separate neural subsystems"[64] with a commonly shared initial analysis of all acoustic input – linguistic, musical or other – in the primary cortex and a subsequent distinguished further processing according to the nature of the signal, with pitch being processed in the right prefrontal cortex and phonetics in the left hemisphere Broca's area.

A less investigated phenomenon, the ability of non-linguistic, musical signals to trigger semantic representations in the brain could be shown by Koelsch et al.[65] In pursuing the question of whether music can "activate brain mechanisms related to the processing of semantic meaning"[66], the authors employed e.g. dissonant music comprising a very small pitch range to represent the word "narrowness" or Beethoven's symphonies to represent the word "hero" and succeeded in demonstrating "that both music and language can prime the meaning of a word, and that music can, like language, determine physiological indices of semantic processing"[67].

The use of music in the context of verbal memory and learning enhancement is not only a basic concept of language-learning strategies such as the suggestopedic approach but has also been examined in comparative studies among children and adults with and without musical education. The suggestopedic approach of language learning includes music for several purposes, two of which are the evocation of a

58 cf. Koelsch et al. (2002)
59 Patel and Peretz (1997)
60 ibid.
61 ibid.
62 ibid.
63 cf. Zatorre et al. (1992)
64 ibid.
65 Koelsch et al. (2004)
66 ibid.
67 ibid.

relaxed but alert state of mind in the recipient, i.e. the learner, and the activation of emotional processes which are to be linked with the newly learned material and thus more deeply rooted in memory.[68] This approach however can prove ineffective or even counterproductive for learners with too much expertise in the field of music. "As in the case of suggestopedic foreign language instruction where the learner is also an experienced music listener, the simultaneous presentation of didactic material and music occasionally causes distraction and / or resistance, hence producing a negative, suggestive effect."[69] Two studies on the potential enhancement of verbal and visual memory through music instruction were able to reveal positive results for verbal memory enhancement in children and in adults after having received music instruction.[70] Chan, Ho and Cheung demonstrated that "adults who received music training before the age of 12 have a better memory for spoken words than those who did not" [71]. Ho, Cheung and Chan confirmed these results for children stating that "Children with music training demonstrated better verbal but not visual memory than those without such training" and went on to examine the long-term effects of music instruction on verbal memory. In a further study on the same subjects after a year's time, those children who had continued their music instruction were able to further improve their verbal memory whereas those children who had stopped their music instruction after three months did not improve their verbal memory any further but were still able to retain their level of verbal memory management previously achieved during their three-month-long instruction in music. However, the authors were able to show an upper limit of verbal memory enhancement in observing the effect that "the longer the duration of music training, the less the improvement in verbal memory tends to be"[72].

The plurality and diversity of studies aimed at the investigation of parallels between language and music processing, production and memorising stress the interconnectivity of strategies and processes involved in the management of both domains. While some shared processes in the perception and production of music and language have already been demonstrated, other seeming parallels still remain unexplained. Without doubt, though, it can be stated that "'music' and 'language' are not independent mental faculties but labels for complex sets of processes, some of which are shared and some different"[73].

68 cf. Brislan (1990)
69 ibid.
70 cf. Ho, Cheung and Chan (2003); Chan, Ho and Cheung (1998)
71 Chan, Ho and Cheung (1998)
72 Ho et al. (2003)
73 Patel and Peretz (1997)

3 Sound-Discrimination Abilities – Their Role in Speech Perception and Language Learning

Sound-discrimination abilities, or auditory discriminative abilities, are in their very general form the competence of distinguishing among acoustic signals or, as Gordon-Brannan and Weiss phrased it, a "[p]rocess of distinguishing among various sounds that may be speech or nonspeech sounds"[74]. In addition to the separation into different domains of application for sound-discrimination abilities, such as language situations, music-receptive situations, noise perception, etc., sound-discrimination abilities can be further subdivided into single abilities. Warren suggests a division into the ability to discriminate loudness, the ability to discriminate phonemes and the ability to discriminate musical sounds.[75]

Sound-loudness discrimination abilities are largely of interest in physical contexts, e.g. in the study of the distinguishability of different degrees of loudness, which can be tested by the "Weber fraction for sound pressure (the proportion by which the pressure of a sound must be different from that of a standard in order for the difference to be detected 50% of the time [...])"[76].

Phoneme-discrimination abilities are the human competence of distinguishing among isolated speech-sounds important for the formation of larger meaning-carrying entities. This ability, as will be discussed in chapter 3.2 below, is universal at birth but specialises towards a distinguishability between language-specifically relevant phonemic contrasts very early in infancy. The ability to identify single phonemes from the general speech flow is considered a curiosity due to the fact that it is impossible to identify the aurally perceived signal in the actual acoustic waveform. This phenomenon has become known as the "lack of invariance problem"[77]. Appelbaum explains that "there is no simple mapping between units of phonetic structure and units of acoustic structure. A single phonetic segment is often realized by different acoustic signals and a single acoustic property may specify different consonants in different phonetic contexts."[78] Coren, Ward and Enns[79] break this phenomenon down into three different indications: a) single phonemes in the speech flow are perceived with physically non-existent pauses between the single speech sounds, b) no injective translation between single perceived phonemes and clearly identifiable acoustic segments is possible and c) the problem of "acoustic-phonetic invariance, the notion that there must be some constant set of acoustic features associated with each perceived phoneme"[80], which means that e.g. "the acoustic set for d [exemplary sound] depends on the context [...] rather than a specific set of invariant acoustic features"[81].

74 Gordon-Brannan and Weiss (2007)
75 cf. Warren (1978)
76 Coren, Ward and Enns (2004)
77 cf. e.g. Appelbaum (1996); Coren, Ward and Enns (2004); Pisoni and Sawush (1975)
78 Appelbaum (1996)
79 Coren, Ward and Enns (2004)
80 ibid.
81 ibid.

Musical sound-discrimination abilities seem a very wide-spread category in this context since they are, again, further divisible into smaller entities of musical sound-discrimination abilities, i.e. the ability to discriminate pitch, tempo, dynamics, harmonic structures, rhythmic structures and melodic structures. These subcategories of musical sound-discrimination abilities will be discussed in chapter 5.1.1 below.

Sound-discrimination abilities play an essential role for the primary purpose of speech perception, i.e. the deduction of conveyed meaning from a speech signal. Whereas loudness-discrimination abilities play only a marginal role for the intelligibility of speech, phoneme-discrimination abilities are of essential importance for both speech perception and speech production. Gordon-Brannan and Weiss noted in the context of the treatment of articulatory disorders that "[i]ndividuals with deviant articulation / phonology seem to have poorer speech perception ability"[82]. Thus, treatment of articulatory disorders does not only focus on the training of speech production but also on the basis of the problem, i.e. the differentiability between phonemically unequal speech sounds.

Theories on the processes involved in speech perception are manifold and include, for example, the motor theory of speech perception, the cohort theory, the trace model of speech recognition and many others. The motor theory of speech perception includes an active speech-production aspect in the process of speech perception assuming that every listener is also a speaker and thus, according to this theory, perception and recognition are only fully achieved by the passive involvement of speech-production mechanisms in the process of speech perception.[83] The cohort theory claims that aurally perceived speech signals are analysed immediately from the perception of the first phonemic information reaching the ear in order to activate the set of words, or cohort of meaningful entities, matching the initially perceived phonemic information. This process is repeated on the reception of every further piece of phonemic information until the cohort of possible words is reduced to a single item and thus recognition has been achieved.[84] The trace model of speech recognition is based on a similar assumption of activation but divides acoustic processing into three different levels: the feature level, the phoneme level and the word level. By activating the first level, all levels are simultaneously addressed and work on a highly interconnected basis including the revision of previously formed hypotheses on possible word input.[85]

While differing in various aspects, such as the active and the passive predominance of perception processing or the order and direction of processes, many theories share the idea of the role of phonemic processing in the course of processes involved in speech perception. After an immediate analysis of the acoustic features of an incoming signal, which is often considered to happen automatically rather than consciously, phonemic processing takes place as a first step of conscious speech processing. This prominent position in the course of speech perception and

82 Gordon-Brannan and Weiss (2007)

83 cf. e.g. Libermann and Cooper (1963); Jusczyk and Luce (2002); Coren, Ward and Enns (2004); Pisoni and Sawush (1975)

84 cf. e.g. Marslen-Wilson and Welsh (1978); Jusczyk and Luce (2002); Coren, Ward and Enns (2004)

85 cf. e.g. McClelland and Elman (1986); Jusczyk and Luce (2002); Coren, Ward and Enns (2004)

word recognition stresses the importance of phoneme-discrimination abilities for the process of speech perception.

3.1 The Role of Sound-Discrimination Abilities in Foreign-Language Learning

Sound-discrimination abilities play an important role in the acquisition and the learning of a foreign language. While loudness-discrimination abilities do not play a role in the sense of discriminating between different levels of loudness, the loudness factor does play an important role in the perception of foreign language along with other factors influencing the perception of a foreign language to a different extent than the perception of a recipient's mother tongue, in the way that successful foreign-language perception and understanding is considerably more distortion-prone and more reliant on an adequate speech volume than first-language perception.[86] Phoneme-discrimination abilities certainly play a central role in the ability to correctly perceive speech signals in a foreign language and are thus essential for the processes of both language learning and language acquisition. Musical sound-discrimination abilities are not thought to play an immediate role in the learning of foreign languages at first sight, an assumption this thesis will hopefully be able to revise.

Phoneme-discrimination abilities in normally hearing adults without any articulation disorders is generally focused on the respective first language's set of phonemic contrasts.[87] The development of phonemic perception and differentiability from early infancy to adulthood will be discussed in chapter 3.2 below. Adults' phoneme-discrimination abilities in foreign languages depend on the discrepancy between the phonemic material forming the learner's first language and the set of phonemes relevant for the foreign language to be learned. Best divided these discrepancies into five different categories of varying difficulty.[88] Discrimination between two non-native phonemes recognised as the same native phoneme and thus representing a phonetic difference which is inexistent in the learner's first language is considered extremely difficult. Discrimination between non-native phonemes which are similar to two different native phonemes, on the other hand, is considered to be easily manageable. Also the discrimination between two non-native phonemes, one of which bears a strong resemblance to a native phoneme whereas the other would be attributed to the same phonemic category of the native language while being notably less similar to the native phoneme, is a distinction classified as feasible. The distinction of speech sounds dissimilar to any of the already known phonemes is considered extremely difficult, whereas the distinction of one dissimilar phoneme and a phoneme similar to a native phoneme should be easily manageable. In the case of foreign-language phonemes which are not identified as actual speech sounds by the learner, the grade of difficulty depends on the phonemes' similarity.[89]

86 cf. e.g. Coren (2004)
87 cf. e.g. Best (1999); Anderson (2003); Werker (1991)
88 cf. Best (1993), Best (1995)
89 cf. eg. Best (1993); Best (1995); Anderson and Morgan (2003)

Success or failure in the discrimination of phonemic differences inexistent in the learner's first language or other previously learned languages does not only depend on the nature of the phonemes themselves but also on the time interval between the perception of the two phonemes. In a study on native English speakers' discrimination ability between two phonemes used contrastively in Hindi but not in English, Werker and Logan were able to show that, whereas the contrast remained undetectable at an inter-stimulus interval of 1500 msec, phoneme discrimination was actually successful at an inter-stimulus interval of 250 msec.[90] Phonemic contrasts specific to the foreign language being learned and not existent in the learner's first or other previously learned languages, however, will most certainly not occur in immediate succession in real-life language situations.

3.2 Sound Discrimination in the Context of the Critical Age Theory for Language Learning

The critical age theory for language acquisition, also known as the critical period hypothesis for language learning, assumes an age window in which language learning has to be initiated in order to be accomplished at all.[91] This age window opens around the age of 2 and closes around the age of 12 and, according to Lenneberg, is limited by "physical immaturity"[92] on the one side and by the "loss of flexibility for cerebral reorganization"[93] on the other. Lenneberg substantiates his claim for a decline of language acquisition abilities by the onset of puberty with electro-chemical changes in the brain up to the age of 10 to 12 years on the one hand and the lateralisation of brain functions up to early puberty on the other hand. Up to the closing of this age window, the brain exhibits the great plasticity necessary for the acquisition of an ability as complex as language.

Singleton contradicts Lenneberg's theory of physical immaturity limiting the language-acquisition process until the age of 2 by stating that "[i]t seems unlikely [...] that there is a particular point in a child's post-natal development where language acquisition can be said to truly begin."[94] Later studies have been able to show that the accustomisation of infants to the language they perceive and thus early language-acquisition processes take place much earlier than initially believed.[95]

Apparent differences between child and adult learners of foreign languages raise the question to what extent the critical age theory is adaptable for second or further language learning. According to Lenneberg, second languages have to be actively studied by learners beyond the age of 12 since "automatic acquisition from mere exposure seems to disappear after this age"[96]. Later studies on immigrants produced contrasting results in favour of better achievement on the part of adult learners on the one hand and in favour of better achievement on the part of pre-

90 cf. Werker and Logan (1985)
91 cf. Lenneberg (1967)
92 ibid.
93 ibid.
94 Singleton (1989)
95 cf. e.g. Werker (1991); Anderson and Morgan (2003)
96 Lenneberg (1967)

pubescent learners on the other hand. Johnson and Newport explain that "[t]his apparent contradiction is resolved when one separates performance in the early stages of learning from eventual attainment in the language."[97] The learning strategies applied by pre-pubescent language learners acquiring language in a steady but slow way differ to a great extent from those applied by adult learners including greater experience in rule-based learning and larger general knowledge. This preliminarily constitutes an advantage for the adult learner over the young learner, a situation which is reversed after a certain time of exposure and amount of input. Singleton summarised the differing learning strategies and the generally poorer ultimate attainment of older language learners in different theories covering the "decreasing sharpness of the senses" in older learners, with special reference to hearing, resulting in the inability to correctly discriminate among non-native phonemes or the interference of first-language habits and rules with the learning of a further language.[98] In this context, Singleton states that "the younger learner is more efficient at acquiring a second language because he or she has accumulated fewer habits to stand in his or her way"[99]. Brain maturity as well as cognitive maturity are further examples of different predispositions in young and old foreign-language learners. Due to declining brain plasticity and lateralisation of phonemic processing in the left hemisphere in late language learners, the younger learner is at an advantage, whereas the adult learner is privileged in terms of cognitive maturity, beneficial for the acquisition of new vocabulary as merely new labels for already known concepts for adult learners while comprising the entire concept learning for very young learners. The acquisition of second-language grammar constitutes another advantage for adult learners, who generally have a better understanding of and a better memory for rule systems.

The critical age theory, at first sight, does seem to prove applicable in terms of phonology. Two phenomena are of interest in this context: a) "While adults are often hampered by their ability to identify or discriminate phones that are not used contrastively in the phonological system of their language(s), young infants do not show such language-specific effects."[100] and b) "Foreign accents cannot be overcome easily after puberty."[101] The second phenomenon seems closely related to the first one in terms of the ability to discriminate and identify a phoneme being a precondition to actively producing it. Moyer explains the difficulty in adult learners' phonology learning in the target language with an "age-related decline in motor control over articulatory organs"[102] on the productive side and a "reduced sensitivity to specific phones that are not members of his [the learner's] L1 [first language] environment"[103] on the perceptive side. In fact, this specialisation and accustomisation to the first language's set of phonemes happens at a very early age.[104] Anderson and Morgan point out that "[i]nfants under six months are able to discriminate native and non-native consonant contrasts equally well, but as they

97 Johnson and Newport (1981)
98 cf. Singleton (1989)
99 ibid.
100 Anderson and Morgan (2003)
101 Lenneberg (1967)
102 Moyer (2004)
103 ibid.
104 cf. e.g. Anderson and Morgan (2003); Werker (1991)

learn the phonological systems of their native language, this ability declines"[105] and "[b]y the end of the first year, infants, like adults, fail to discriminate many non-native contrasts"[106]. This phonological focus towards the learner's first language, however, is not irreversible. Wang and Kuhl point out that "auditory training studies have successfully trained adult listeners to better distinguish non-native sounds"[107], which coincides with Anderson and Morgan's conviction that "adults' ability to discriminate certain non-native contrasts can improve with training"[108]. In terms of production of non-native phonemes by adult foreign-language learners, Moyer constitutes one possible source of error in the perception of target-language phonemes similar to first-language phonemes being highly prone to confusion: "[i]n cases of close similarity, the learner is likely to perceive the two counterpart sounds as equivalent, and establish a close, but inaccurate, target for the new sound"[109]. However, whereas ultimate attainment of phonology in the target language is clearly more often realised by learners with a pre-pubescent age of onset, "with sufficient experience and exposure, adult second language (L2) learners can authentically perceive or produce novel L2 sounds which have no native language (L1) phonemic counterparts"[110]. Wang and Kuhl imply further factors in this statement, namely experience and exposure hinting at the possibility of the age factor being only one of many influential factors for attainment in second-language acquisition. Moyer sums this up by pointing out that "attainment in L2 phonology is highly variable, probably because of multiple factors of experience that exert differential influence across learners and learning situations"[111].

As stated above, sound-discrimination abilities with respect to phonology are developed and specialised towards the perceived language's set of phonemes at a very early stage during the first year after birth. However, phoneme-discrimination abilities are not a fixed value after their first development but can be trained to include additional phonemic differences to those used in the learner's first language. This leads Wang to the conclusion in reference to Lenneberg's critical age theory introduced above that "L2 learning is probably not a strictly timed developmental process with rigid cut-off periods, as claimed by the CPH [critical period hypothesis], but is rather a function of experience and exposure"[112], coinciding with Moyer's statement that "language acquisition relies on more than just neurological processes"[113].

105 Anderson and Morgan (2003)
106 ibid.
107 Wang and Kuhl (2003)
108 Anderson and Morgan (2003)
109 Moyer (2004)
110 Wang and Kuhl (2003)
111 Moyer (2004)
112 Wang and Kuhl (2003)
113 Moyer (2004)

4 Methods for the Testing of Sound-Discrimination Abilities

The testing of human sound-discrimination abilities, in particular speech-sound discrimination abilities, dates back as far as 1931 with Travis and Rasmus[114] pioneering in the examination of differences in the speech-sound discrimination skills of subjects ranging in age from junior primary school to adulthood. Whereas sound-discrimination ability tests generally refer to tests of any kind of acoustical input including the testing of speech-sound, noise and music, the focus in this context will be kept on speech-sound discrimination, only taking into account a few cross-domain studies which have made use of musical sound-discrimination tests.[115]

This chapter will present a brief overview of previously developed and applied methods for the testing of human sound-discrimination abilities, which have a broad history in clinical treatment of hearing impairment on the one hand and diagnostics of reading difficulties in beginning readers on the other hand. Studies and tests on sound discrimination in foreign languages are rare and sound discrimination in foreign languages unknown to the subjects appears only marginally tested. This, in addition to the fact that the majority of previous testing methods have been developed and designed to match the requirements of very young subjects, necessitated the development of a new speech-sound discrimination test to meet the requirements of the present study as will be described in detail in chapter 4.2 below.

4.1 Previously Applied Sound-Discrimination Tests

Testing in the field of human sound-discrimination abilities, also referred to as aural discrimination skills[116] or auditory discrimination skills[117], with its history of almost eight decades, has been carried out with a variety of intentions and not in all cases for the mere purpose of determining selected groups of subjects' sound-discrimination abilities.

This chapter is not intended to give an extensive overview of all previously applied tests of this manner, but shall serve instead as a brief introduction to the different fields of application by presenting some examples for the respective fields. In addition to the general testing of human sound-discrimination abilities, which can be subdivided into the testing of subjects' individual progress in sound-discrimination ability over a period of time[118] and the comparison of different test groups' sound-discrimination abilities[119], and the obvious application of sound-discrimination tests in

114 Travis and Rasmus (1931)
115 For further information on the testing of sound-discrimination in music, refer to chapter 5.1.1 below.
116 cf. Gromko et al. (2009)
117 cf. Wepman (1958); Bradley (1972)
118 cf. Mansur (1950); Pronovost and Dumbleton (1953); Wepman (1958); Snow and Hoefnagel-Höhle (1979)
119 cf. Templin (1943); Templin (1957); Danhauer, Crawford and Edgerton (1984)

the diagnostics of and research in the domain of hearing impairment[120], tests of this kind have also been carried out to survey possible correlations between sound-discrimination abilities and reading abilities[121], pronunciation and articulation abilities[122] and verbal memory[123]. Further studies employing sound-discrimination testing have been concerned e.g. with the preference of information input in either acoustical or visual form over the respective other[124].

Studies on the individual development of sound-discrimination abilities as carried out by Mansur[125], Pronovost and Dumbleton[126] and Wepman[127] generally aim at the investigation of children's sound-discrimination abilities in their mother tongue, i.e. English in the case of the aforementioned studies. Studies dealing with the testing of sound discrimination in foreign language acquisition, as issued e.g. by Snow and Hoefnagel-Höhle[128], are scarcer and cover a broader age range of their subjects, also exploring the sound-discrimination abilities of adults.

Pronovost and Dumbleton tested the sound-discrimination abilities of 434 first-grade school children by means of a revised version of the original Mansur Test[129] developed in the course of a Master thesis, the revised version of which became known as the Boston University Speech Sound Discrimination Test.[130] The test consisted of monosyllabic minimal pairs of words, which could be unambiguously displayed as pictures. The subjects were asked to choose from a set of three picture pairs whether one of the words was heard twice or both words were heard. The original test by Mansur also used a fourth option requesting the order of the heard words, which was omitted in the revised version due to the fact that "many young children have visual reversals", which were not the target of testing in this context and thus "may have affected the results on the Mansur test"[131]. Fifty percent of the presented test items made use of two identical words and fifty percent constituted minimal pairs, which differed in either primacy, mid or recency position. All test items were read out to the subjects by the test administrator.

The auditory discrimination test developed by Wepman[132] for the application with five- through eight-year old children consists of 40 pairs of monosyllabic English words, which the subjects have to be classy as being identical or different. Wepman included ten pairs of identical words and 30 minimal pairs in the test. In evaluating a subject's results, a distinction was made between the two types of possible errors, namely the subject falsely classifying two identical words as different and the subject falsely classifying two different words as identical. A subject is considered to have failed the test when too many errors have been made, according to a list of maximum error amounts corresponding to the subject's age.

---

120 cf. Bradley (1972); Finnegan (1974); Bochner et al. (1997)
121 cf. Cabot (1968); Anvari et al. (2002)
122 cf. Travis and Rasmus (1931) and Sherman and Geith (1967)
123 cf. Gromko et al. (2009)
124 cf. Camp (1970)
125 Mansur (1950)
126 Pronovost and Dumbleton (1953)
127 Wepman (1958)
128 Snow and Hoefnagel-Höhle (1979)
129 cf. Mansur (1950)
130 cf. Merleau-Ponty (1981)
131 Pronovost and Dumbleton (1953)
132 Wepman (1958)

Snow and Hoefnagel-Höhle tested 51 English-speaking immigrants to the Netherlands learning Dutch "naturally, with no formal training" [133] for their progress in discriminating Dutch sounds which are not distinctive phonemes in English in three separate tests at an interval of four to five months, with the first test carried out six months after the subjects' arrival in the Netherlands. The subjects were subdivided into three different age groups, which consisted of 19 three- to seven-year olds, 22 eight- to fifteen-year olds and 11 adults. Only one part of the battery of ten subtests was concerned with auditory discrimination of phonemes. The subjects were confronted with minimal pairs differing in phonemes which are not differentiated among in English and were asked to point to the respective picture of the word they believed to have heard. In the course of the study, two differently developing skills became obvious, with grammatical skills and phonological skills improving independently at different speeds and to different degrees in the individual subjects. Auditory discrimination was found to correlate with varying factors of language learning at the different test stages, first appearing entirely independent of pronunciation, then correlating with progress in vocabulary and grammar skills still seemingly independent of pronunciation and finally, in the third and last test, "pronunciation and auditory discrimination correlated highly and formed one factor, suggesting that perceptual ability had become the limiting factor in pronunciation skill"[134]. The correlation between auditory discrimination and pronunciation has been investigated before by Travis and Rasmus[135] and Sherman and Geith[136] in the context of native-language use and will be introduced below.

The comparison of different test groups' sound-discrimination abilities was in the centre of attention for Templin[137] and Danhauer, Crawford and Edgerton[138] with the latter expanding into the field of comparison between native speakers of different languages.

Templin developed two similar tests carried out with children of different age groups, intending to survey differences in children's sound-discrimination abilities according to their age, their sex and their socio-economic background. The first test, developed in 1943, was carried out with three-, four- and five-year old children, who were asked to classify 59 minimal pairs of monosyllabic English words displayed as pictures as either "same" or "different". Differences in phonemes occurred in primacy, mid and recency position. Templin was able to show that children from a stable socio-economic background performed better on the sound-discrimination test than children from underprivileged socio-economic backgrounds. In a second test, developed in 1957 for the examination of six-, seven- and eight-year olds' sound-discrimination abilities, Templin made use of nonsense syllables consisting of an initial consonant and a final vowel or vice versa, again asking the subjects to decide whether the two presented syllables had been the same or different. This test revealed better results for older children than for younger ones. Within the different age groups, children from a good socio-economic background performed better than

133 Snow and Hoefnagel-Höhle (1979)
134 ibid.
135 Travis and Rasmus (1931)
136 Sherman and Geith (1967)
137 Templin (1943); Templin (1957)
138 Danhauer, Crawford and Edgerton (1984)

children from an underprivileged socio-economic background and girls made fewer mistakes than boys.

Danhauer et al. tested the applicability of a nonsense-syllable test of sound discrimination for native speakers of Spanish, English and bilingual Spanish and English speakers. Ten adult English speakers, ten mostly adult Spanish speakers and nine adult bilinguals were asked to repeat invented consonant-vowel-consonant-vowel disyllabic words, first presented at different levels of volume through a loudspeaker, then by the test administrator. Even though the test made use of invented nonsense words, it could not produce the same results for native Spanish speakers as it did for native English speakers. Only the results achieved by the English speakers and those achieved by the bilingual Spanish and English speakers were comparable.

The testing of sound-discrimination abilities appears of special importance in diagnostics and research in the field of hearing impairment. Three exemplary studies in this field were concerned with the examination of the sound-discrimination abilities of mentally challenged subjects[139] and of subjects with cleft palates[140] and the testing of subjects' sound-discrimination abilities as a form of diagnostics of the subjects' type of hearing impairment[141]. Further examples of diagnostic tests from the German-speaking area are *Heidelberger Lautdifferenzierungstest (H-LAD)*[142], *Bremer Lautdiskriminationstest (BLDT)*[143] and *Lautunterscheidungs-test für Vorschulkinder (LUT)*[144].

Bradley[145] examined the sound-discrimination abilities of 60 mentally challenged subjects, 30 of which had been diagnosed with auditory motor deficits, also referred to as word-sound deafness, and 30 of which had been diagnosed with auditory autonomic deficits, also referred to as word-meaning deafness. The test employed in this study was a composite test comprising elements of the Templin Picture Sound Discrimination Test and the Wepman Auditory Discrimination Test described above and additional tasks requiring the subjects to repeat 30 test items after the test administrator. Subjects with auditory motor deficits were found to achieve notably lower scores in all sound-discrimination tests than subjects with auditory autonomic deficits.

In a test of speech-sound discrimination abilities of 32 eight-year old male subjects, half of which had a cleft palate, Finnegan[146] compared the auditory discrimination skills of subjects with and without a cleft palate, of cleft-palate subjects with and without impaired hearing abilities and of subjects with and without velopharyngeal incompetence. The sound-discrimination test applied in this study comprised six different task types, all of which consisted of pairs of consonant-vowel-consonant monosyllables containing phonemes the subjects were unable to pronounce properly. The initial and final consonant of the first syllable were always the same and the contrasts between the two presented syllables were either an

139 cf. Bradley (1972)
140 cf. Finnegan (1974)
141 cf. Bochner et al. (1997)
142 cf. Brunner, Dierks and Seibert (2005)
143 cf. Niemeyer (1970)
144 cf. Fried (1980)
145 Bradley (1972)
146 Finnegan (1974)

alteration of the initial consonant only, the final consonant only or both consonants. As a further degree of difficulty, the altered consonants were replaced by their respective voiced or voiceless equivalent. Finnegan was able to show that non-cleft palate subjects made fewer mistakes than cleft-palate subjects, eight-year olds made fewer mistakes than seven-year olds within both groups, subjects without any form of hearing impairment unsurprisingly made fewer mistakes than subjects with hearing impairments, subjects with velopharyngeal incompetency made fewer mistakes than subjects without velopharyngeal incompetency and subjects with both middle ear pathology and velopharyngeal incompetency made the most mistakes.

In 1997, Bochner et al.[147] were among the first to employ a computerised testing method to survey the remaining sound-discrimination abilities of 73 young deaf adults. The subjects were asked to compare a set of four sentences to a target sentence classifying them as identical to or different from the target sentence. The progress in the computerised testing version lies in the program's ability to adapt to the specific performance level of the individual subjects individually selecting the next more difficult, same level or less difficult test item according to the subjects' performance on previous test items. Since the testing program ends as soon as there are no appropriate test items left in terms of difficulty level, the test can be of different length for different subjects. In contrast to other sound-discrimination tests, this test makes use of real-life language situations asking the subjects to discriminate between complete sentences rather than isolated syllables. The authors conclude that "scores on the SSPDT[148] provide diagnostic / analytic information about examinees' ability to process acoustic and phonetic dimensions of speech"[149].

In 1968, Cabot[150] examined the relation between primary school children's reading abilities and their auditory discrimination abilities. 149 first graders and 182 second through fourth graders were asked to classify 38 pairs of two-phoneme monosyllables consisting of an initial consonant phoneme and a subsequent vowel phoneme as either identical or different. A standardised reading test was used to determine the subjects' reading abilities. The auditory discrimination test was found to be a reliable predictor of failure in reading abilities with a low sound-discrimination ability correlating with a low reading performance. This led the author to the conclusion that the ability to discriminate between speech sounds is "a necessary though not a sufficient condition for reading"[151].

More recent studies on the correlation between sound-discrimination and reading abilities are closely interlinked with the discrimination of musical sounds in addition to the discrimination of speech sounds. By means of the Bentley test of musical ability described in context with the introduction of musicality tests in chapter 5.1.1 below and a standardised reading test, Barwick et al. were able to show "positive relations between tonal memory and reading age, and between chord analysis and reading age"[152]. Also Lamb and Gregory found out "that discrimination of musical sounds is related to reading performance"[153]. In accordance with the

147 Bochner et al. (1997)
148 Speech Sound Pattern Discrimination Test
149 Bochner et al. (1997)
150 Cabot (1968)
151 ibid.
152 Barwick et al. (1989)
153 Lamb and Gregory (1993)

above-stated results, Anvari et al.[154] found a close relationship between music perception and phonological awareness as well as early reading development in four- and five-year old children.

The possible relations between speech-sound discrimination abilities and pronunciation abilities are probably among the first aspects examined in the history of sound-discrimination testing. As early as in 1931, Travis and Rasmus[155] carried out a series of studies examining the sound-discrimination abilities of subjects with and without functional disorders of articulation ranging from junior primary school children to adult subjects. The authors showed that subjects with speech disorders made notably more mistakes in a speech-sound discrimination test asking the subjects to decide whether two contrasting pairs of English speech sounds were identical or different. In accordance with the authors' hypothesis, most mistakes were made by subjects with articulatory difficulties with precisely those phonemes which could not be pronounced correctly by the respective subjects.

Sherman and Geith[156] later made use of the Templin test of auditory discrimination described above in order to examine the relation between kindergarten children's speech-sound discrimination abilities and their articulation skills. The authors were able to show that children with good speech-sound discrimination skills achieved notably better results in a test of their articulation skills than children with poor speech-sound discrimination abilities.

More specialised studies making use of sound-discrimination tests have been carried out by Camp[157] to investigate the preference of either acoustic or visual information input over the respective other and by Gromko et al.[158] to analyse the relationship between children's memory for tones, numbers and nonsense words and their sound-discrimination ability. Camp made use of the wide-spread word-pair method asking the subjects to decide whether the second item of the heard pair was the same as or different from the first. Differences in the monosyllabic English words occurred in either primacy, mid or recency position and were presented to the kindergarten and first-grade school children in the form of illustrations. Camp was able to show a preference for either visual or acoustical input over the respective other for at least 25% of the tested subjects. Gomko et al. on the other hand applied a reproductive kind of sound-discrimination test asking the tested first- through third-grade school children to reproduce 30 heard sets of three syllables, numbers and tones. The authors showed a positive correlation between the subjects' sound-discrimination abilities and their ability to reproduce numbers. Correlations between sound-discrimination abilities and the ability to recall tones and syllables could be observed but failed to prove statistically significant.

154 Anvari et al. (2002)
155 Travis and Rasmus (1931)
156 Sherman and Geith (1967)
157 Camp (1970)
158 Gromko et al. (2009)

4.2 The Necessity for a New Testing Method

As the context of the present study is very different from the general contexts of application for sound-discrimination tests, it is not possible to use previously applied and established testing methods for the fields of examination and the tested subjects in the present study.

As shown above, the majority of sound-discrimination tests have been designed for the testing of children and are not suitable for application with adults. Furthermore, the tests introduced above are based on languages known to the tested subjects, if not testing isolated phonemes or nonsense syllables, as e.g. in the case of the tests developed by Travis and Rasmus[159] or Templin[160].

All of the above-described testing methods, with the exception of the test applied by Bochner et al.[161] surveying the processing of complete sentences and the tests by Danhauer et al.[162] and Anvari et al.[163] making use of di- and multisyllabic words, are limited to the discrimination of monosyllables. In addition to the isolation of the tested sounds, which certainly is a legitimate method in the testing of hearing impairment, pronunciation deficits or reading difficulties, the discrimination between the tested sounds was almost in all cases limited to the decision of whether the two sounds were identical or different.

Thus, the present study, aiming at the investigation of adult subjects' sound-discrimination abilities in a de facto existent language, which is not isolated from its actual contextual meaning in its presentation to the subjects but is unknown to them, required the development of a new testing method.

4.2.1 Requirements of a Sound-Discrimination Test for the Purposes of the Present Study

As already indicated above, the requirements for a sound-discrimination test in the present study are very different from other previously developed and applied sound-discrimination tests, which to a great extent are applied in the field of medical diagnostics or the examination of learning difficulties in children.

The present study, aimed at the investigation of the sound-discrimination abilities of normally hearing adult subjects without any learning difficulties, requires a test suitable for application with adults and capable of determining adequately distinguishable degrees of the tested abilities. Thus, the test battery has to include an adequate number of different degrees of difficulty within the test items as well as different kinds of tasks for the subjects to solve rather than the mere decision of whether two consecutive pieces of acoustical information are the same or different. Furthermore, it is of extreme importance for the test items to occur in a natural

159 Travis and Rasmus (1931)
160 Templin (1943)
161 Bochner et al. (1997)
162 Danhauer, Crawford and Edgerton (1984)
163 Anvari et al. (2002)

context carrying actual meaning. The meaning itself, of course, is not relevant for the discrimination of sounds, but presenting the form of input in a natural-like context by using meaning-carrying utterances of a native speaker is of great importance for the determination of whether strange sounds can be recognised and differentiated among when heard in their natural surrounding.

In addition to the content-related reasons for a new test, there were also practical ones leading to the decision to use a computer-based test to be carried out on the internet. The tested subjects were from different parts of Germany and volunteered at different times to take part in the study. A computer-based testing method made it possible for the subjects to individually carry out the tests from their homes at times most suitable for them, allowing for a relaxed test atmosphere. From the test administrator's point of view, conducting the test via the internet meant a direct access to and the undelayed further processing of all gathered data.

4.2.2 Testing of Adults' Sound-Discrimination Abilities in an Unknown Foreign Language

The test of adults' sound-discrimination abilities in an unknown foreign language developed and applied in the context of the present study consists of two separate online multiple-choice tests to be carried out with an interim interval of two weeks. The foreign language exemplary examined in this context is Finnish, a phonetic language and thus well suited for the present testing purposes. The language applied in this context had to meet the requirement of being a phonetic language in order to enable the subjects, as novices to the sound of the language, to match the aural input of heard sounds with the visual input of written characters presented to them in the course of the test. Furthermore, Finnish was chosen as the language for testing because of the high probability of finding a large number of subjects inexperienced in this language in contrast to other phonetic languages such as Latin. The inexperience in the language to be tested is a crucial requirement to be met by the subjects in order to guarantee an equal starting level for all subjects. A further criterion supporting the choice of Finnish in this context is the fact that the Finnish alphabet does not contain any letters unknown to the German-speaking subjects of the study. Ö/ö and Ä/ä, the only extra characters in the Finnish alphabet, are used in German as well and did thus not present any problems to the subjects. Whereas largely an independent language of original terms for expressions, such as for example computer, which is called *tietokone* (knowledge machine), Finnish does also include loanwords from other languages, which might be easy for German-speaking subjects to guess. Since the present test is aimed at the subjects' sound-discrimination abilities and does not want to venture into the domain of semantics, loanwords such as *mikrofoni* (microphone), *gangsteri* (gangster) or *bokseri* (boxer) have been omitted from the words, phrases and sentences used in the course of this test. All audio files applied as listening examples for the test were recorded with a native Finnish speaker.

Each test consists of 62 questions with nine grades of difficulty and eight different question types. In a first question type, the students are asked to tell how many words they believe to have heard in a sentence. This question type is available for every grade of difficulty with grade-one sentences consisting of three mono- or disyllabic words, grade-two sentences of three tri- or quadrisyllabic words, grade-three sentences of three words with five or more syllables, grade-four sentences of four mono- or disyllabic words, grade-five sentences of four tri- or quadrisyllabic words, grade-six sentences of four words with five or more syllables, grade-seven sentences of five or more mono- or disyllabic words, grade-eight sentences of five or more tri- or quadrisyllabic words and grade-nine sentences of five or more words with five or more syllables. The subjects are to choose their answer from a selection of four answer options in the case of the lower-grade questions and five answer options in the case of the upper-grade questions. For example, the sentence *Oli kiva nähdä sinut taas.* (It was nice to see you again.), a grade-seven sentence with five mono- and disyllabic words, is played while the answer options of three words, four words, five words and six words are displayed.

In a second question type, the subjects are asked to tell which word they heard at a certain slot within the sentence. This question type delivers a graphic representation of the sentence in the form of underscores representing the single words of the sentence and an X marking the slot of interest for the respective question. This kind of question occurs in every grade of difficulty. The answer options are equal to the words occurring in the sentence and thus the number of answer options depends on the grade of difficulty with three options for grades one through three, four options for grades four through six and five or more options for grades seven through nine. For example, the sentence *Isännän vieraat saapuivat myöhemmin.* (The guests of the landlord arrived later.) is used as a grade-five question in the context of looking for the word filling the third slot of the sentence with *isännän*, *myöhemmin*, *saapuivat* and *vierat* as answer options occurring in alphabetic order. For sentences containing words beginning with an umlaut, e.g. *äiti* (mother), the alphabetic order of German, which is familiar to the subjects, has been applied rather than the Finnish alphabetic order. For the present example of the word *äiti*, the initial "ä" is treated as a normal "a" for sorting purposes whereas it would be treated as an extra character after Z in Finnish. (A screenshot of the described question as occurring in the online test is shown in figure 4-1 below.)

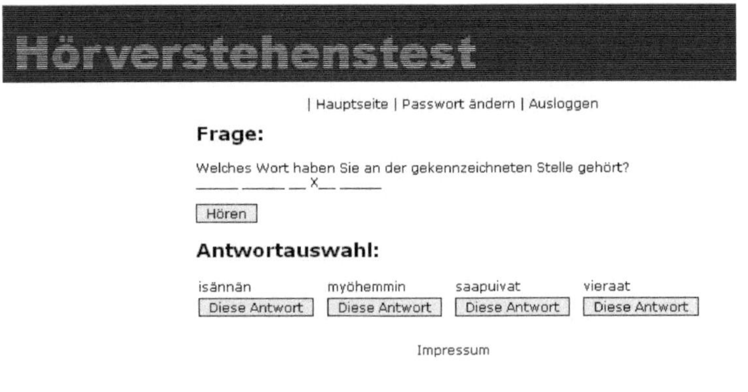

figure 4-1: question on the identification of a word in a certain slot of the sentence

A further task type asks the subjects to identify a heard word from a set of four or five written words. The words to compare differ in similarity and in word length for the different grades of difficulty. Grade-one questions consist of mono- or disyllabic words, grade-two questions of tri- or quadrisyllabic words, grade-three questions of words with five or more syllables constituting the words sought after with additional answer options on the basis of the correct answers, with however one syllable more or less. For example in the grade-one question applied in this context, the audio file for *maassa* (in the country) was presented together with the written answer options of *maa* (country), *maassa* (in the country), *maassakin* (in the country, too), *maassako* (In the country?) and *maassani* (in my country) in alphabetic order. Grade-four through grade-six questions are based on the differentiation principle between single exchanged consonants or vowels with grade-four words being mono- or disyllabic, grade-five words tri- or quadrisyllabic and grade-six words consisting of five or more syllables. For example the grade-four question in this context presented the audio file of the disyllabic word *turva* (protection) together with the written answer options of *turha* (in vain), *turma* (accident), *turpa* (mouth – for animals or in rude language), *turta* (numb) and *turva* (protection) in alphabetic order. Grade-seven questions focus on the differentiation between single and double vowels and consonants in disyllabic words. Grades eight and nine do not exist for this question type due to the lack of sufficient multisyllabic words at this degree of similarity. For example the audio file of the word rumaa (ugly – in the partitive form of the word)[164] is issued together with the written answer options of ruma (ugly), rumaa (ugly – in the partitive form of the word), ruuma (cargo compartment) and ruumaa (cargo compartment – in the partitive form of the word).

The fourth question type applied in the course of the sound-discrimination test is focused on the recognition of the location of a written word in a heard sentence. The number of answer options to choose from depends on the sentence length and thus the grade of difficulty. For example the audio file of the sentence *Voitteko odottaa huonessa.* (Please wait in the room.)[165] is presented in the context of looking for the word *huonessa* (in the room) and occurs together with the three answer options a) in first position, b) in second position and c) in third position. There are no deceptive answer options such as "in fourth position" for a three-word sentence. The number of answer options, sentence and word lengths for the different grades of difficulty are equal to those described in the context of the second question type above.

The fifth question type is similar to the above-described third type asking the subjects to identify a heard word from a set of four or five written words. In this context, however, the task is inverted in the sense that the subjects are asked to identify a written word out of a set of four or five independently playable audio files of similar words. The words are similar to the degrees explained in the context of the above-mentioned question type. For example, when looking for the word *siika* (whitefish), the audio files of the words *sika* (pig), *sikaa* (pig – in the partitive form

164 *Partitiivi* (partitive) is one of the fifteen cases in Finnish. It is used to express an undefined quantity of something and occurs with nouns as well as with their describing adjectives as in the context described above. It is comparable to the partitive use of *de* in French, such as in *Je bois du lait.* (I drink milk.), which also expresses an undefined quantity of its subsequent noun.

165 in polite form of address equal to the German *Sie* as opposed to *du*

of the word) and *siikaa* (whitefish – in the partitive form of the word) are presented as wrong answer options together with the audio file of the word *siika* (whitefish).

The sixth question type aims at testing the subjects' ability to remember word orders. The audio file of a Finnish sentence depending on the respective grade of difficulty in length and word complexity, as described above, is presented together with a number of drop-down menus equal to the amount of words in the respective sentence. Each drop-down menu contains an alphabetically ordered list of all words occurring in the sentence constituting three equal drop-down menus for the questions of grades one through three, four equal drop-down menus for grades four through six and five or more equal drop-down menus for grades seven through nine. For example the grade-nine question making use of the audio file of the sentence *Luonnonsuojelijat varoittivat mahdollisista muuttuvista luonnonilmiöistä.* (The conservationists warned of possibly changed nature phenomena.) includes five equal drop-down menus consisting of *luonnonilmiöistä*, *luonnonsuojelijat*, *mahdollisista*, *muuttuvista* and *varoittivat* in this order with the display fields of all menus initially set to the alphabetically first occurring word *luonnonilmiöistä*. (See figure 4-2 below for a screenshot of this question.) The selections made for the single drop-down menus are not immediately accepted as the subjects' final answers but can be altered until the *Abschicken* (send) button has been clicked.

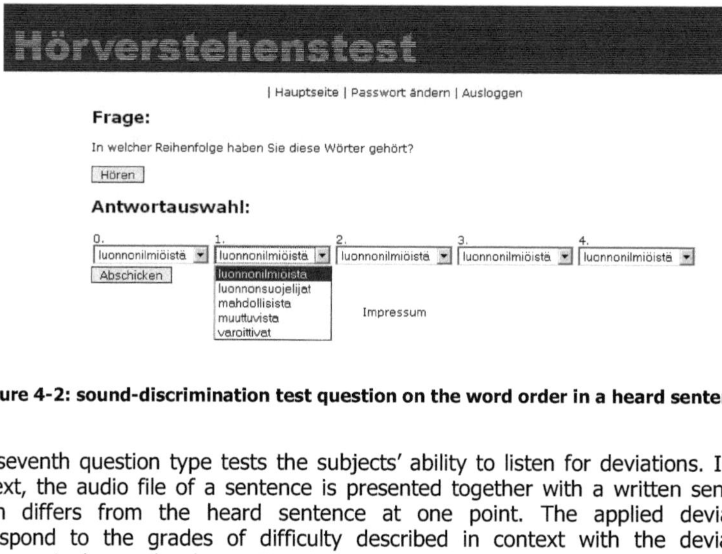

figure 4-2: sound-discrimination test question on the word order in a heard sentence

The seventh question type tests the subjects' ability to listen for deviations. In this context, the audio file of a sentence is presented together with a written sentence which differs from the heard sentence at one point. The applied deviations correspond to the grades of difficulty described in context with the deviations between single words above. To give an example of a grade-five question, the sentence *Koululaiset söivät ranskalaisia perunoita.* (The pupils ate French fries.) is presented as an audio file together with the written answer options of *koululaiset*, *syövät* (eat), *ranskalaisia* and *perunoita* in the order of the sentence.

In a final question type, the subjects are asked to identify a heard sentence from a set of similar written sentences which differ from each other to the above-explained extent. For example, the grade-four question in this context employs the audio file of the sentence *Missä kirjasi nyt on?* (Where is your book now?) and, in addition to the corresponding written sentence, the two sentences *Missä kirjani nyt on?* (Where is my book now?) and *Missä kirjansa nyt on?* (Where is his/her book now?), which are altered by one syllable as has been determined for grade-four through grade-six questions.

To grant comparability, the second test consists of the same questions in the same order as the first test with different words and phrases of the same level of complexity. An alteration with respect to the tested words and phrases is necessary to avoid any potential bias of the subjects towards answers previously chosen during the first examination. For example, for the grade-seven question of the second question type looking for a certain word at a marked slot in the sentence (see figure 4-1 above for a screenshot of this type's grade-five question), the first test employs the sentence *Äiti ei tule tänään koska hän on seiras.* (The mother is not coming today because she is ill.) while the second test makes use of the same amount of words and a similar sentence structure issuing the sentence *Lapsi ei tahdo tulla kotiin koska hän leikkii.* (The child does not want to come home because he/she is playing.). In both questions, the respective word for the third slot in the sentence is being sought.

5 Methods for Testing and Training of Musical Listening Skills

The training of musical listening skills is a major constituent of the present study. Testing and training methods in the field of musical listening skills appear to differentiate between non- or not-yet-musicians and musicians in their choice and characteristics of applied tasks. Whereas the available methods for aural training in music seem to exclusively direct themselves at musicians and learners of instruments, the so-called musicality tests or musical aptitude tests presuppose a not-yet-musician as a potential test taker. This has caused a severe methodology problem for a study in which non-musicians, usually the subjects of the testing side of musical listening skills, shall receive an aural training in music usually designed for musicians. The requirements for a training conception were not fully met by any of the available aural training programs, eight of which are introduced as examples in the following. This necessitated the development of a new training conception meeting all the requirements for aural training in music under the special conditions of the present experiment.

5.1 Previously Available Test and Training Conceptions

5.1.1 Musicality Tests

Musicality tests or tests of musical aptitude are generally directed at non-musicians or not-yet-musicians without any considerable prior knowledge in the field of music practice. The tests are mostly designed to measure children's potential for discrimination between single sounds, sound patterns and sound sequences but have been applied to adult subjects as well. Most of the tests do not claim to be capable of measuring a person's musical aptitude in general but stress the fact that only single elements which are part of musical intelligence are tested.

It is not the purpose of the present subchapter to provide an extensive overview of all musicality tests currently available.[166] However, insight into how musicality tests are structured, what elements of music they use for measuring and what kinds of tasks they employ for the subjects to solve is essential for the development of aural training for non-musicians in the context of the present study as described in chapter 5.2.2 below. For this purpose, the test methods of Bentley[167] and of Seashore[168] shall be briefly introduced and compared.

Both the Measures of Musical Abilities by Bentley and the Measures of Musical Potential by Seashore are tests designed for a classroom situation. Whereas the Bentley test is clearly structured for children as test subjects comprising a total of 60 questions in the four categories of pitch, melody, rhythm and harmony, the Seashore

166 For an overview of tests on musicality and musical aptitude, see Füller (1974).
167 Bentley (1966)
168 Seashore (1960)

test directs itself towards children from age ten up to adults, providing a considerably larger amount of, in total, 260 questions in the categories of pitch, volume, rhythm, tone length, timbre and melody.

The pitch-discrimination questions are similar in both tests with an identical reference tone for every task being a standard 440 Hz tone a^1 in the Bentley test and a 500 Hz tone, a tone between b^1 and c^2, in the Seashore test. Bentley includes identical intervals in his questions, whereas the Seashore answer options only consist of the two choices of a higher or a lower tone. The maximum interval tested with Bentley is a half step, whereas Seashore employs a frequency difference of 17 Hz constituting a 3.5th tone at the applied frequency range. The minimum intervals tested are a 17th tone in the Bentley test and a 28.9th tone in the Seashore test. Other intervals tested are a 2.9th tone, a 4.3rd tone, a 5.1st tone, a 6.4th tone, a 8.5th tone, a 10.2nd tone and a 12.8th tone with Bentley and a 4.9th tone, a 7.3rd tone, a 11.6th tone, a 14.5th tone and a 19.3rd tone with Seashore.

In both the Bentley and the Seashore tests, the subtest questions concerning rhythm consist of rhythmic pairs which are either equal or different. Whereas the Seashore test only issues the two answer options of equal or different, the Bentley test asks the test takers to specify which beat of the second rhythm was different. Bentley applies a wide range of easy to complex rhythmic figures, such as a crotchet, two quavers, a quaver triplet, four semiquavers, a quaver and two semiquavers, two semiquavers and a quaver, a quaver embraced by two semiquavers, a triplet consisting of a crotchet and a quaver, a dotted quaver and a semiquaver and a semiquaver and a dotted quaver, on four beats played at a speed of 72 bpm. The length of Seashore's rhythm tasks, on the other hand, varies from five tones in two-four measure and six tones in three-four measure to seven tones in four-four measure played at a speed of 92 bpm.

The melody tasks for both the Bentley and the Seashore test consist of melody pairs to be compared by the test taker. The second melody always differs from the first melody by one tone. Bentley's melodies consist of five tones whereas the length of Seashore's melodies varies between three, four and five tones. Seashore employs different intervals for the tone alteration in the second melody, whereas the interval difference between Bentley's first and second melody is always either a minor or a major second. Bentley also includes the answer option of the two melodies being equal in case the subject is not able to hear any difference between the two melodies. The ambitus of applied tones is a fifth ranging from d^1 to a^1 with Bentley and one and a half octaves starting from c^1 with Seashore.

The chord-analysis task included in the Bentley test does not have any parallel in the Seashore test. Bentley uses 20 of the 60 test questions on the identification of the number of tones played in a chord with ten diads, eight triads and two four-note chords.

Seashore, on the other hand, includes subtests on volume, tone length and timbre in his musicality test, all of which consist of comparison tasks with tone pairs. The volume tasks range from volume differences of a maximum of 4 dB to a minimum of 0.5 dB played at a constant frequency of 440 Hz. The second tone is always either louder or softer than the reference tone. The tasks concerning tone length also make use of a 440 Hz tone played at different lengths. The difference between the first and the second tone amounts to a maximum of 0.3 seconds and a minimum of 0.05 seconds. The timbre questions are based on the dominance of single overtones over others. The basic tone is located at 180 Hz, a tone between f and f sharp, and within the first five overtones sounding together with the basic tone, the volume of the fourth overtone is raised simultaneously with the volume of the third overtone being lowered. The easiest questions constitute a volume difference of plus 10 dB for the fourth overtone and minus 9.6 dB for the third overtone, whereas the most difficult questions comprise volume changes of plus 4 dB for the fourth overtone and minus 0.7 dB for the third.

5.1.2 Aural Training Programs and Concepts

The methods and concepts for aural training in music are various and, though often largely differing in their modus operandi, they always aim at training the same fields of perception within a piece of music, if admittedly often to different extents. It is not the purpose of this chapter to present an extensive discussion of every method available for aural training in music. However, it is essential to briefly introduce a few exemplary concepts in order to demonstrate the necessity of developing yet a different kind of aural training, which is designed to meet the requirements of aural training in the special context of the present study.

The methods for aural training presently available are largely classifiable into four different conceptions. The classical methods presuppose a classroom situation with a teacher conveying certain hearing strategies to pupils who already have a basic knowledge of music theory and who actively play an instrument. Later developed methods consider the fact that the main learning process in aural training takes place in a self-study situation without a teacher, yet still assume an instrumentalist as a student. By the end of the 1990s and with greater availability and use of computers, musical hearing-training programs were available in the form of computer programs designed for self-study in the context of a general musical and instrumental education. Today, in the age of the internet, musical listening-training is available on numerous websites as well, most of which are designed for the use of already trained musicians with a certain level of previous knowledge in music theory as well as in piano playing.

The teaching conceptions exposited by Quistorp[169] and Mackamul[170] are two examples of the classroom-situation kind of aural training. Quistorp includes additional tasks of singing, clapping and writing music for self training in her otherwise teacher-centred concept, which mainly focuses on dictation tasks. Her concept divides the learning groups into five different levels of competence. Reading and writing music make up a large part of the training tasks. Even the lower grade groups quickly proceed to rather complex musical structures, such as syncopes and 64th note phrases in rhythm training or four- and five-note chords in harmony training. The training fields within this concept comprise rhythm training, interval and melody training and chords and harmony training. Mackamul's school of aural training is designed for small groups of students instructed by a teacher within three different grades of difficulty. The training includes active participation of the students

169 Quistorp (1970)
170 Mackamul (1969)

by singing, clapping and instrumental playing, with reading and writing music being requirements for the participation in an aural training course according to Mackamul. This training concept includes different kinds of tasks besides the usual dictation tasks. The students are further asked to repeat tunes played by the teacher, to analyse tunes played by the teacher, to sing melodies prima vista and to compare written music scores with heard music played by the teacher. This training concept presupposes a certain background knowledge of music theory for all students. The fields of study within this concept include rhythm training, interval and melody listening and reproduction of one-voice and two-voice melodies and harmony training.

The aural training concepts by Kühn[171] and Kaiser[172] are two examples of self-study training. Kaiser, however, introduced a multipurpose conception for self-training on the one hand and for the use in seminars on the other hand. Both Clemens and Kaiser base their listening examples to a large extent on excerpts from known pieces of classical literature. Piano playing, singing, music reading and the knowledge of basic music theory and terminology are presupposed in both training concepts. Whereas Kühn focuses on the training of melody and harmony listening, Kaiser additionally expands his training concept with an extra volume focused on the training of rhythmic figures. Neither pitch nor tempo are among the training fields of Kühn's and Kaiser's conceptions. Lesson timing and answer feedback are only a part of Kaiser's training concept in the case of the classroom application rather than self-study use of the program.

The two examples of computer-based self-study programs briefly introduced in the following are only two of many programs of this kind currently available. Both Auralia[173] and the program by Bendig[174] presuppose a music student or at least the learner of an instrument as a user of the program, assuming knowledge of musical terms to different degrees. Auralia includes a wide selection of help sites accessible throughout the use of the program, providing information on music theory and musical terms and also including listening examples. Bendig, on the other hand, applies alternate terms such as space and time instead of tone length or rhythm and tone height or melody, yet presupposes the knowledge of terms such as augmentation and diminution. Both training concepts do not follow any specific order of tasks but leave it up to the user to decide which field of training and which kind of task to practice at what time. Bendig also leaves the choice of task difficulty, ranging from a to c, up to the user, whereas Auralia, with six different levels of difficulty, makes use of pop-ups suggesting the user continue with the next higher level within the respective training category, though leaving it up to the user to decide whether or not to take the suggested step. Both training programs include active participation tasks such as singing and piano playing. Auralia gives immediate feedback on the user's answers, which in case of the singing tasks, are sung into a microphone and in case of the piano-playing tasks are played via a midi-keyboard. Whereas Auralia evaluates the user's input and gives feedback, the program by Bendig is based on self control and evaluation. Bendig divides his training concept into the three categories of space, i.e. pitch, melodies and harmonies, time, i.e. tone length and

171 Kühn (1983)
172 Kaiser (1998)
173 Rising Software (2003)
174 Bendig (1999)

rhythm, and space – time, i.e. rhythmic melodies, whereas Auralia is divided into the four categories of chords, rhythm, pitch and melody. Both programs do not provide any fixed training times. However, Bendig suggests the user of his program practice for 20 minutes three times a day and Auralia offers the option of presetting a test with a freely selectable number of questions at a selectable level of difficulty. Whereas Bendig's concept, relying on the students to check their own work, does not include any record of tasks previously worked on or answers previously given, Auralia offers the opportunity to view extensive reports on the users' training sessions and progress.

Two of the online aural training programs currently available for self-study via the internet can be found at http://www.musikwissenschaften.de and at http://www.musicians-place.de.[175] Both training concepts primarily aim at tutoring learners of musical instruments, with the musikwissenschaften training presupposing a basic knowledge in piano-playing. Musicians-place focuses on the aural training of intervals, chords and scales including the less common Dorian, Phrygian, Lydian, Mixolydian and Locrian scales while musikwissenschaften aims at the training of intervallic listening and melodies. The typical musicians-place training entity comprises five tasks, which can be freely generated by the user with several presettings, such as downwards or upwards proceeding or simultaneously played intervals, the interval range to be tested, simultaneously played or arpeggiated chords and the inversion of the chords to be tested. After answering the five displayed questions, the user receives a detailed answer overview showing his or her own answers as well as the correct answers for the respective questions. Musikwissenschaften also features individual adjustment of the test contents and difficulty. Intervals can be played successively or simultaneously with a fixed or varying first tone and a higher or lower or varying second tone. The interval range to be tested can be set to a minimum of a third and a maximum of a tenth. Interval tests feature some means of help such as the displaying of the first tone in a score and, if not disabled, also the second tone. The keyboard displayed below the task can be used as an additional help for finding tones. One training module consists of twenty questions with direct answer feedback after every answered question indicating either a correct or an incorrect answer, the latter of which remains uncorrected in this training conception. The melody training is based on imitating atonal melodies played by the program by means of the displayed keyboard. The tones played by the program are additionally displayed in written form in the score displayed above the task.

Whereas teaching methods and training tasks may vary throughout the different conceptions of aural training, the addressee of these conceptions is always a musician or the learner of an instrument. This entails the specific teaching of music theory as well as the practical involvement of the trainee's respective instrument and voice, which is inappropriate for aural training for non-musicians as applied in the present study. An overview of the requirements to be met by the single aural training methods introduced above will be given in chapter 5.2.1 below.

175 The online training conceptions briefly described in this chapter are, as any other internet content, subject to constant changes. All observations in this context are based on the sites' status of November 29th 2008.

5.2 The Necessity for a New Training Method

The aural training conceptions introduced above give a vague idea of the broad variety of aural training programs for musicians and learners of a musical instrument. However, the subjects of the present study, specifically being non-musicians, would not be able to participate in most of the training conceptions described above due to their inexperience in music reading and piano playing and their lack of knowledge of music theory and terminology. Both the practical side of classical aural training and the introduction to music theory are unasked for in the context of the present study focusing on sound-discrimination abilities and thus on pure listening to, as opposed to active participation in, music. Conceptions for the application to non-musicians seem to be present in the form of musicality tests only, rather than actual training. However, this study does not aim to test the subjects' sound-discrimination abilities in music but wants instead to use music as a means of training the subjects' sound-discrimination abilities while testing is carried out in the field of foreign language perception. All this called for a new concept making use of task types resembling those of the musicality tests described in chapter 5.1.1 above together with training fields resembling those of the aural training programs described in chapter 5.1.2 above.

5.2.1 Requirements of an Aural Training for the Purposes of the Present Study

An aural training program in music for the special context of the present study does not only have to meet the requirement of being suitable for novices to the field of music practice and especially to aural training in music but also has to focus on the aspect of pure listening training rather than the teaching of music theory usually inseparably interwoven with the general aural training conceptions as described above. Even though the training applied in the present context does not need to consist of extensive course work for a long period of time, relatively quick progress towards different levels of difficulty for the tasks to be worked on is essential in the present context. Music theory and music terminology are neither to be presupposed nor to be taught, yet the aural training should include the training fields of melody, rhythm, harmony, pitch and tempo, employing only audio files and graphic representations in addition to the question text. The pitch tasks should not include any typical teaching of interval determination but focus on the aspect of different tunings of one and the same tone. Practical tasks such as singing or piano playing should not be part of the training, which is instead focused on the trainees' listening abilities rather than practical skills which are not previously known by the subjects and shall not be taught in this context. The listening tasks presented by the program, however, should vary and draw the trainee's attention towards different elements of the respective listening examples including comparison tasks, anticipation tasks and tasks on the graphic representation of heard material which is not presented in the form of common notation but in a form generally intelligible for non-musicians without any knowledge in music reading. The training concept to be applied has to meet the requirement of being a self-study concept with a certain degree of tutoring in order not to distract the user of the program with external non-training elements such as keeping the training time in mind or checking for correct answers from external material. In the context of minimising possible distractions from the actual training, the application of musical material previously unknown to the user of the program is of extreme importance in order to keep the subjects' attention on the tasks to work on rather than potentially arising questions as to where he or she may know the respective listening example from.

Table 5-a below gives an overview of the required elements for an aural training to be applied in the context of the present study including the aural training conceptions described in chapter 5.1.2.

	different levels of difficulty	melody training	rhythm training	harmony training	pitch training	tempo training	no music theory	no instrumental practice	no theoretic terms	no practical tasks	different task types	self-study concept	answer feedback	lesson timing	unknown music examples
Quistorp (1970)	X	X	X	X	-	-	-	-	-	-	X	-	X	X	X
Mackamul (1969)	X	X	X	X	-	-	-	-	-	-	X	-	X	X	-
Kühn (1983)	X	X	-	X	-	-	-	-	-	-	X	X	-	-	-
Kaiser (1998)	X	X	X	X	-	-	-	-	-	-	-	X	-	-	-
Bendig (1999)	X	X	X	X	-	-	-	-	-	-	X	X	-	-	-
Auralia (2002)	X	X	X	X	X	-	-	-	-	-	X	X	X	-	X
Ehlert (2008)	X	X	-	-	-	-	-	-	-	-	-	X	X	-	X
Sedlmeier (2008)	X	-	-	X	-	-	-	X	-	X	-	X	X	-	X

table 5-a: overview of the requirements met by the aural training conceptions introduced in chapter 5.1.2

As the table shows, none of the above-introduced training conceptions meets all of the requirements essential for an aural training for non-musicians. Especially the non-theoretical aspect is not met by any of the conceptions introduced above. As a consequence of the lack of an aural training program suitable for self-study application of non-musicians, the aural training ToSCA[176] was developed and applied in the context of this study.

176 Training of Sound Contrasting Abilities

5.2.2 ToSCA – Training of Sound-Contrasting Abilities, the Training Program Applied in the Course of the Present Study

The computer-based music program for the training of sound-discrimination abilities, henceforth referred to as ToSCA, has been developed particularly for use in and the requirements of the present study by the author of this thesis. It is a musical hearing-training program which consciously excludes any kind of music terminology and which does not teach the concepts of music theory underlying the classical music of the Western world usually introduced in the prevalent musical hearing-training programs. The special focus of ToSCA is on the training of contrasting, recognition and anticipation of single sounds, sound sequences and sound patterns in the form of music.

ToSCA is programmed for fourteen consecutive training units of fifteen minutes daily for a period of two weeks.[177] The single sessions are automatically terminated by the program after fifteen minutes of training and it is not possible to re-start the program on the same day, in order to prevent any potential shortening of the two-week training period. For any unforeseen events during the fifteen minutes of training, the program is equipped with a break function, which can pause the program so no time is lost in case of unforeseen events during the subjects' training time. All buttons except for the re-start button are disabled during the state of pause so that it is not possible to play the listening examples and extend the time for selecting an answer for the displayed question. All listening examples are playable twice in order to allow a second comparison and not more than twice in order to prevent a direct comparison between the given listening example and the answer options to choose from. The play buttons are equipped with an indication of how often the single listening examples are still playable counting backwards from "2x" to "0x" in order to allow for the user to keep an overview of the playability of the single listening examples, which otherwise might become confusing with up to five examples to click and listen to. Every answer option is equipped with a solve button, which turns either green or red after clicking in order to let the trainee know whether or not his or her choice was correct. In order to achieve a teaching effect, which is essential for the training purposes of ToSCA, all answer options are highlighted with red colour for the wrong answers and green colour for the correct answer, as shown in figure 5-3 below.

177 The duration of the training has been determined based on reasons of organisation and in order to keep the work load in reasonable bounds for the voluntary subjects, who do not receive any money for their work. The results of the study will have to show whether this relatively short training will prove sufficient for an obvious and measurable effect.

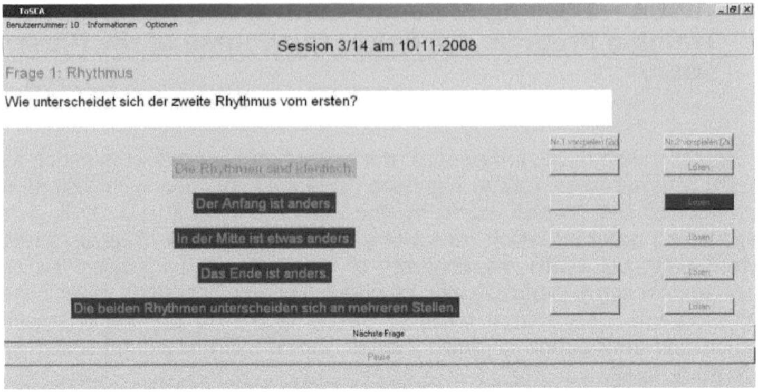

figure 5-3: ToSCA interface after clicking a wrong solve button[178]

The program covers five different fields of training: pitch, tempo, melody, rhythm and harmony, with each field of training further subdivided into five different levels of difficulty, which can be reached independently of the respective other fields in order to guarantee a subject-individual training at the trainee's own speed of learning and according to their individual skills. The entire program is based on six different types of questions aimed at the sound-discrimination, -recognition and -anticipation skills to be trained: a) the direct comparison between two sounds, b) the recognition of a given sound from a selection of others, c) the identification of the one sound from a selection of sounds which differs the most from the first heard sound, d) the selection of the most fitting sound for the conclusion of an unfinished melody or harmony sequence, e) the identification of the one sound from a selection of sounds which would not lead an unfinished melody or harmony sequence back to a musically logical ending and f) the matching of the heard sound sequences with a selection of graphical representations of sound sequences.[179] The question types as well as the fields of training occur in random order and are automatically selected by the program from a large number of possible questions and a wide range of possible wrong answers to display in addition to the correct answers. The structure of question types, fields of training and levels of difficulty is visualised in figure 5-4 below. The specified question types, however, do not occur in all fields of training depending on the characteristics of the respective field, i.e. there are no sound, sound sequence and sound pattern anticipation questions concerning the identification of the only musically logical conclusion of an unfinished musical entity or the exclusion of one musically illogical conclusion of an unfinished musical entity in the fields of pitch, tempo and rhythm. The fields of pitch and tempo do not lead to any specifically necessary conclusion per se and can thus be omitted. The field of rhythm could have been included in the tasks of logical conclusions, but, since it is

178 The interface language of ToSCA is German since the program was written for and applied to German-speaking subjects only.

179 All question types also contain tasks concerning sound sequences and sound patterns rather than single sounds.

much more ambiguous than the fields of melody and harmony, which are clearly aiming at and asking for a certain ending, it has also been omitted in order to avoid confusion among the subjects to be trained. The second and last exception is the transfer task of matching a heard sound pattern with its graphical equivalent, which does not occur for tempo and harmony questions.

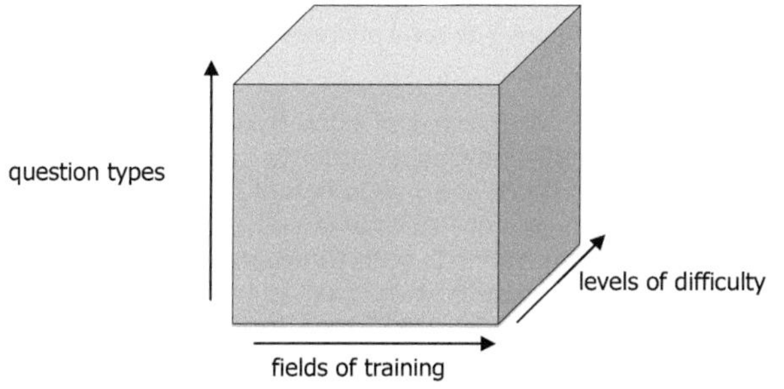

figure 5-4: structural concept of ToSCA

The score assignment for questions answered by the trainee works in both directions in order to avoid any possible progress to the next higher level by pure guessing. One point per correctly answered question is added to the total score in the respective training field while one point is deducted for each incorrectly answered question. However, it is not possible to obtain a negative score so the trainee could never get into the position of first having to answer a certain number of questions correctly before receiving any credit for his answers again. For the information of the trainee and for motivational purposes, the current scores of all five training fields are always visible in graphical form at the bottom of the program window. A green bar either moves one step further to the right for a correctly answered question or one step back to the left for an incorrectly answered question in the respective field of training. In total, five bars, one below the other, indicate the current progress within the single levels and thus allow for a direct comparison between the trainee's performance in the individual training fields[180]. The next higher level is reached after the accumulation of 18 points respectively. These thresholds were established after previous testing of the program and according to the training duration and the expected performance of the subjects previously untrained in music. The maximum score of 90 points, which can be achieved at the end of level five, cannot be exceeded, in order to prevent the situation of a trainee being able to incorrectly answer an undefined number of questions without being downgraded to the fourth level.

180 see figure 5-3

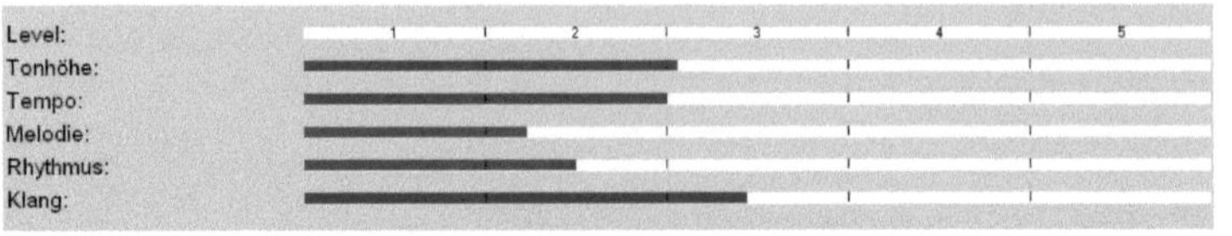

figure 5-5: level overview in ToSCA

The direct-comparison task in the field of pitch training consists of two consecutive tones which are independently playable in order to allow the trainee to memorize the single tones for as long as he or she needs before hearing the respective reference tone.[181] Three types of answers are selectable with this kind of task asking how the second tone is different from the first: both tones are equally high, it is higher and it is lower. The difference between the two tones to be compared is a quarter tone for level one, an 8th tone for level two, a 16th tone for level three, a 32nd tone for level four and a 64th tone for the final level five. The tone range for the pitch questions is subdivided into three different pitch ranges of a perfect fifth plus the level-specific deviation in both upward and downward direction. The different ranges are separated by an octave minus the level-specific deviation. The tasks are randomly chosen from the three different frequency ranges, i.e. the low frequencies ranging from F to c, the mid frequencies ranging from c^1 to g^1 and the high frequencies ranging from g^2 to d^3. In order to avoid a very unlikely but nevertheless possible habituation to certain frequencies and to provide a greater range of frequency comparisons, the program does not only choose the pure tones as basic tones for the pitch comparison, but also their down-tuned and up-tuned versions. Thus the program randomly chooses questions from a selection of 45 possible tasks for level one, 135 possible tasks for level two, 855 possible questions for level three, 1,215 possible tasks for level four and 1,395 possible tasks for level five[182]. The differences perceivable for musically untrained subjects were tested among nine musically untrained subjects in a pre-study, which resulted in all nine subjects generally being able to differentiate between quarter tones while the amount of correct answers decreased for the comparison between less different tones. The test was carried out for the intervals of a quarter tone, a 6th tone, an 8th tone, a 16th tone, a 32nd tone, a 64th tone and a 128th tone within the low-, mid- and high-frequency tone ranges described above. Whereas most subjects were still able to answer questions on the 32nd-tone intervals correctly, the results for the 64th-tone questions already appeared to be random and led to the assumption that the subjects were only guessing by that interval. This is why there are no questions on intervals of 128th tones included in ToSCA. Furthermore, since all nine subjects were still able to correctly answer the mid-range 8th-tone questions, the 6th-tone questions were left out of the final program as well.

181 All listening examples are played in a piano sound, except for the examples of the rhythmic training categories, which are played by a low tom and a high-mid tom.

182 The amount of possible questions is stated without consideration of their additionally occurring permutations. Therefore the effective number of possible questions is much higher, since the single answer options are not generated in a specific order by the program.

The recognition tasks in the field of pitch training are based on the same tone ranges and level-specific deviations as the comparison tasks described above. The program randomly chooses a question out of a selection of 15 possible questions for level one, 45 possible questions for level two, 285 possible questions for level three, 405 possible questions for level four and 465 possible questions for level five. The trainee is asked to recognise a given reference tone out of a set of three tones to choose from. One of the selection tones equals the reference tone, one is higher by the interval of the previously described level-specific deviation and one is lower by the interval of the level-specific deviation. Once again the number of possible questions within the single levels of this kind of task depends on the set tone range and the tone intervals asked for in the respective levels. Each tone for the use of the pitch training tasks is available in 33 versions for the program to choose and pose questions from: one pure version, 16 down-tuned versions in 64th-note steps and 16 up-tuned versions in 64th-note steps with the sixteenth 64th-note step being a quarter tone off the pure tone in either direction respectively. To give an example from the second level, there are three questions possible employing the tone d^1: looking for the pure tone d^1 with the eighth 64th step downwards and the eighth 64th step upwards as additional wrong answers, looking for the eighth 64th step downwards with the pure tone and the sixteenth 64th step downwards as additional wrong answers or looking for the eighth 64th step upwards with the pure tone and the sixteenth 64th step upwards as additional wrong answers. All intervals amount to the level-specific deviation of an 8th tone for level two, so with three possible questions per tone in a five-tone range and three tone areas, there are 45 possible questions for the program to choose from in this level.

In a third question type within the training field of pitch, the trainee is asked to identify the tone, the height of which differs the most from the reference tone. The program randomly poses questions from a selection of 24 possible questions for level one, 30 possible questions for level two, 90 possible questions for level three, 570 possible questions for level four and 810 possible questions for level five. The program puts out three answers to choose from, with one answer being the level-specific interval higher than the reference tone, one answer being the level-specific interval lower and one answer being either the level-specific deviation higher than the already higher tone or the level-specific deviation lower than the lower tone, which amounts to an interval twice as wide as the level-specific deviation for the correct answer being sought. This may, at first glance, seem like a contradiction to the intervals set for each level, but on closer inspection, it becomes clear that the level-specific deviations are still kept in this kind of task. To give an example from the third level, the interval which is being trained in this level is a 16th tone. The program may present f^1 as a reference tone and, as possible answers to choose from, its by a 16th note down-tuned version, its by a 16th note up-tuned version and its by an 8th note, and thus two 16th notes, up-tuned version. Thus, the smallest interval to differentiate between always remains a 16th tone, whereas it would be only half as wide, if the most different tone sought after already were the interval of a 16th tone off the reference tone, so the other two examples to choose from would have to be in between the reference tone and its by a 16th tone down-tuned or up-tuned version. The trainee, however, is not yet asked to recognise the difference between intervals closer than a 16th note at the stage of level three.

The last question type within the pitch training category concerns the identification of the reference sounds in the form of graphical representations. The graphical representation task in this training category is rather simple compared to the graphical representation tasks for melodies and rhythms, which are to be explained in more detail below. However, graphical-representation tasks were included in the training categories wherever possible, since this kind of transfer between acoustic and optic input is also asked for in the identification of written language from heard language in the course of the sound-discrimination tests described in chapter 5.1. The program randomly chooses from a selection of 105 possible questions for level one, 135 possible questions for level two, 1,125 possible questions for level three, 1,305 possible questions for level four and 1,395 possible questions for level five. In level five, for example, the by fourteen 64th tones down-tuned version of f may be put out as a first reference tone to be compared with the by thirteen 64th tones down-tuned version of f as a second reference tone, being a 64th tone higher than the first reference tone. The trainee was confronted with three different graphics to choose from: one displaying two consecutive bars of the same height, one displaying the second bar higher than the preceding bar and one displaying the first bar higher than the subsequent bar, as shown in figure 5-6 below. The two reference tones are independently playable in order to give the trainee enough time to memorise the first reference tone or even to listen to the first tone twice before listening to the second reference tone.

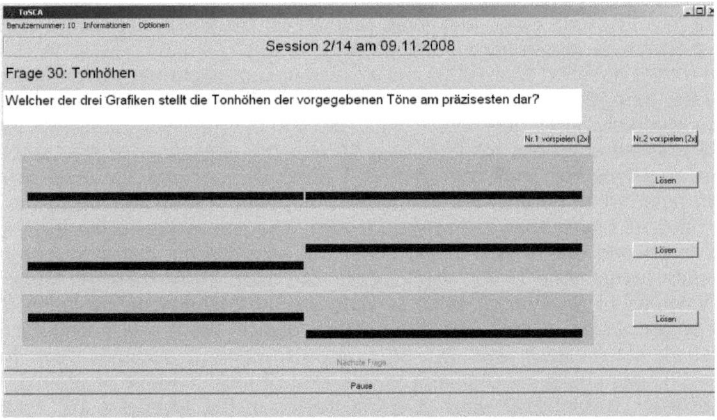

figure 5-6: transfer question within pitch training

The training category for tempo comprises the three question types concerning comparison, recognition and the identification of the listening example which differs the most from the reference example. In order not to distract the trainee from focusing on the tempo rather than other elements of the listening example, only rhythmic pieces are employed for the questions of this training field. The rhythms used in this context are taken from the rhythm-training category of ToSCA, which differ in their complexity according to the levels they are composed for. Once again, in order not to distract the trainee from the original task, only simple rhythms of level one are applied in this category. The general tempo of the rhythm tasks is 100 bpm with 50 percent of the rhythms being of a straight four-four measure and 50 percent being of a three-four measure, both of which are applied for the tempo-training category. To acoustically mark the first beat of the bar, which is important for the distinction between single bars and between three-four measure and four-four measure examples, the first beat of every bar is played by a low tom whereas all other beats are played by a high-mid tom. The different characteristics of the level-specific rhythms are mostly irrelevant for this training category and thus will be described in the context of the rhythm-training category below in this chapter.

The direct-comparison task within the tempo-training of ToSCA issues a first and a second reference rhythm which do not differ in their rhythmical structure but only in their tempo from a very clear difference of 30 bpm, resulting in 130 bpm and 70 bpm rhythms for level one to a rather narrow difference of 5 bpm, resulting in 105 bpm and 95 bpm rhythms for level five. Level two asked the trainee to differentiate between 20 bpm resulting in 120 bpm and 80 bpm rhythms, whereas level three asks for a differentiation between 15 bpm, resulting in 115 bpm and 85 bpm rhythms and level four asks the trainee to differentiate between 10 bpm, resulting in 110 bpm and 90 bpm rhythms. While the rhythms and possible questions are randomly chosen for this kind of task, the answer options always remain the same. The trainee is asked to decide whether the rhythms are either equally fast or whether the second rhythm is faster or slower than the first. For the two reference rhythms, the program randomly chooses questions to pose from a selection of 36 possible questions for each level. As an example of a level-three question within this category and question type, ToSCA may put out rhythm A in its original 100 bpm version as a first rhythm and rhythm A in its accelerated 115 bpm version as a second rhythm awaiting the answer "The second rhythm is faster than the first."

The recognition task within tempo training is based on the same rhythmic patterns applied for the question type described above as well as on the same tempo deviations of 30 bpm for level one to 5 bpm for level five. ToSCA randomly picks a reference rhythm in its original tempo of 100 bpm and additionally chooses three matching answer options based on the reference rhythm: one version which is equal to the reference rhythm, one version which is faster by the level-specific deviation, and one version which is slower by the level-specific deviation of, e.g. 15 bpm for level three. The program poses questions out of twelve possible tasks per level.

The pitch-training task of identifying the rhythm which differs the most from the reference rhythm does not only employ the level-specific faster and slower versions of the single rhythms described above but also versions which are the level-specific tempo deviation slower than the already slower versions and versions of the level-specific tempo deviation faster than the already faster versions. These tasks, similarly to the pitch-training tasks of the same question type, make use of listening examples which deviate twice as much from their original reference examples as determined in the level specifications. However, once again, the trainee is only supposed to be able to differentiate between tempi within the deviation range of the respective level. In this context, the already slower and the already faster versions of the original reference tempo are to be seen as the reference tempi for the further accelerated and decelerated tempo versions. Any further subdivision into tempo versions between the reference tempo and its respective faster or slower version as another opportunity to create tasks for this question type would anticipate the training difficulties of higher levels, which is unasked for in this context. The program poses questions from a selection of 24 possible tasks for each level respectively, employing the original 100 bpm tempo versions as reference examples and the respective level-specifically deviating, faster and slower versions together with either the twice-accelerated or the twice-decelerated tempo versions as answer options.

The training field of melody is the one training category employing all occurring question types. This, however, does not mean that the melody category is being trained more than the other categories since the single categories of pitch, tempo, melody, rhythm and harmony are randomly selected by the program for every new question. The higher number of question types in this category only offers a wider variety of possible questions for the program to pose. The melodies are level specific and become more complex with each higher level, starting from two bars of crotchets with a closing minim for level one and ending with two bars of semiquavers with a closing crotchet for level five.[183] All melodies are played at a tempo of 100 bpm in four-four time without any rhythmic variations in order not to distract the trainee from the task of dealing with the melodic progression rather than with any other element of the music. The keys of the listening examples vary with an equal division between minor and major key tasks and no key reoccurring with a second melody of the same level. Level-two melodies consist of four bars of crotchets with a closing minim, level-three melodies of two bars of quavers with a closing crotchet and level-four melodies of four bars of quavers with a closing crotchet. It may be argued that level-two and level-three as well as level-four and level-five melodies train listening examples of the same lengths in terms of the number of notes occurring per melody. However, whereas the number of notes stays the same, the duration of the listening examples of the respective higher level is only half as long as for the preceding level meaning the trainee is to remember twice as much information per bar as before. The higher levels additionally differ from the lower ones in their complexity, i.e. in their ambitus and in their melody-progression intervals. Whereas melodies of the lower levels mainly progress in seconds and thirds without the use of many larger intervals and only comprise a small ambitus of no more than one octave, melodies of the higher levels frequently employ fourths, fifths or sixths in their melody progression, clearly exceeding the octave range in their ambitus.

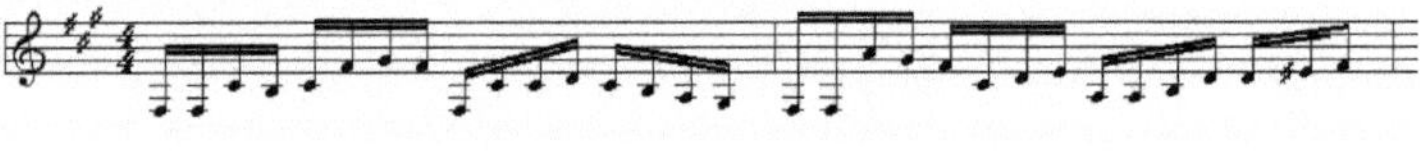

figure 5-7: example of a level-five melody

For the comparison task in the field of melody training, the trainee is confronted with two similar melodies, which are independently playable for the same reasons of the subjects' individual memorising strategies explained in context with the comparison tasks in the categories of pitch and tempo training above. The trainee is asked to decide how the second melody is different from the first with four answer options to

183 See figure 5-5 for an example of a level-five melody.

choose from: the beginning is different, the middle is different, the end is different or both melodies are identical. The extent to which the two melodies are different is level dependent and decreases with each next higher level, starting from a whole bar of difference in level one constituting 50 percent of the listening example and progressing to a crotchet-length difference in level five constituting 12.5 percent of the melody. The substituted parts in the deviating melodies do not necessarily have to consist of 100 percent different tones. A single tone may be equal to the melody's original version. However, according to Gestalt theory[184], it will be perceived differently in a different context and, being a single identical tone, will not be recognised as a part of the reference melody but instead as a part of the new, altered version occurring in a different melodic progression context. Figure 5-8 shows an example of a level-two reference melody with its respective altered-beginning version sharing one common initial tone.

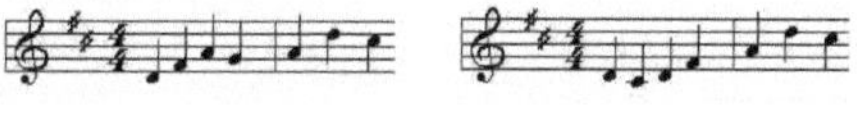

figure 5-8: altered melody beginning for level-two comparison tasks

The program poses questions from a set of 48 possible tasks per level at a random order. Each reference melody has a specific counterpart with either an altered beginning, an altered middle part or an altered ending. As a result, the same reference melody may reoccur in a different context and with a different correct solution.

The recognition task in the category of melody training consists of one reference melody and four comparative melodies as answer options, one of which is identical to the reference melody. The program randomly chooses three additional melodies which are similar to the reference melody and only differ in either their beginning, their middle part or their ending by the level-specific deviation lengths. The program randomly chooses questions out of a selection of 1,260 possible questions per level, placing the answer options in random order.

The melody-training task of identifying the listening example which differs the most from the reference melody makes use of a second set of altered melodies consisting of versions which either deviate more than the level-specific extent for levels two through five or less than the level-specific extent for level one. Level one is treated exceptionally in this context in order to keep the task easy for the beginning level. The normal altered melody versions for level one already differ in most tones from their reference versions due to the short listening examples of only two bars employed in level one. The altered melody versions of the extra level-one melody set only differ in one single tone from their reference melodies, forming the wrong answers for this question type, whereas the extra set of altered melodies for level two up to level five differing by more than the previously altered melody versions are used as correct answers in this context. The additionally altered versions differ from their reference melodies by two bars and thus 50 percent of the total melody length for level-two tasks, by one and a half bars and thus 37.5 percent for

184 For more information on Gestalt theory, refer to e.g. Ehrenfels 1988, Thomas 1990 and Wertheimer 1969.

level-three tasks, by one bar and thus 25 percent for level-four tasks and by half a bar and thus 25 percent for level-five tasks. The program randomly displays tasks out of a selection of 192 possible questions for level one and 144 possible tasks for levels two through five, always displaying three wrong answers along with one correct answer. The wrong answers consist of either the reference melody itself, the altered-beginning, altered-middle or altered-end version deviating to the respective level-specific extent for level one and deviating by more than the determined level-specific difference for levels two through five.

The melody- and harmony-training specific tasks of identifying the one melody or harmony which does not form a logical solution for a melody or harmony beginning make use of two further sets of melody variations. All of the above-described melodies end on the respective listening example's tonic. In the context of this question type, the reference melody does not end on the tonic but on the fifth forming the antecedent of and thus opening a musical phrase. The trainee is asked to identify the one consequent out of four answer options which does not lead the phrase back to its tonic.[185] In addition to the above-introduced set of melody versions ending on the fifth, there are further melody versions employed which differ in their ending according to the melody's level. The melody variations presented as consequents in level one end on the augmented unison, the minor third, the tritone, the minor sixth or the minor seventh for major melodies and on the augmented unision, the major third, the tritone, the major sixth or the major seventh for minor melodies, all ending tones not being part of the respective melody's key. Other occurring wrong consequent endings are the third introduced from below, the fourth introduced from below, the fifth introduced from above, the sixth introduced from above, the sixth introduced from below, the seventh introduced from above and the seventh introduced from below for levels two and three and the third introduced from above, the fourth introduced from above and the fifth introduced from below for levels four and five. The altered melody versions in their level-specific and their long versions as well as the original reference melodies described above in context with the other question types employed for melody training, which all end on the tonic, are used as possible wrong answers in the context of looking for the consequent not leading its respective antecedent back to a logical ending. The program randomly poses questions out of a selection of 2,100 possible tasks for level one, 2,940 possible tasks for levels two and three and 1,260 possible tasks for levels four and five.

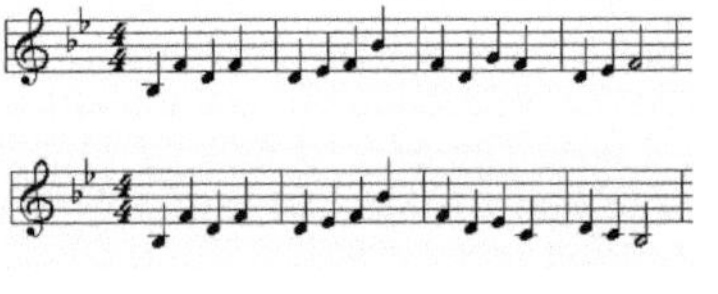

figure 5-9: level-two melody example of an antecedent ending on the fifth and a matching consequent ending on the tonic

185 For an example of an antecedent-type reference melody with a matching consequent, see figure 5-7.

The inverted task of identifying the only consequent which guides the reference melody back to its tonic is another part of the melody-category training. For this question type, the above-described sets of altered melody versions are employed with inverted functions. The consequent versions ending on the tonic are employed as correct answer options and the consequent versions ending on the level-specific different scale or non-scale steps are employed as additional wrong answers. The reference melodies consist of the same set of antecedents ending on the fifth as for the above-described question type. In the context of this part of the training, the program has a selection of 840 possible questions for level one, 2,940 possible questions for levels two and three and 84 possible questions for levels four and five at its disposal.

For reasons of memory capacity, the program does not include any picture files in context with the transfer tasks. The graphics used for the training of visual recognition of heard melodies are automatically generated and put out together with the respective questions by the program.[186] All previously described consequents ending on the tonic are employed as reference melodies. Their respective altered versions in their extreme and in their normal versions are used as models for the wrong-answer graphics put out together with the correct graphic equivalent of the reference melody. The program poses questions from a selection of 1,260 possible tasks for each level. Figure 5-10 shows an example task in which the melody version with an altered middle part is used as a reference melody (the second graphic in the example). The first graphic, as a wrong answer option, is the graphic equivalent of the melody's version with an extra long altered middle part and the third graphic, as the other wrong answer option, is the graphic equivalent of the melody's version with an extra long altered ending.

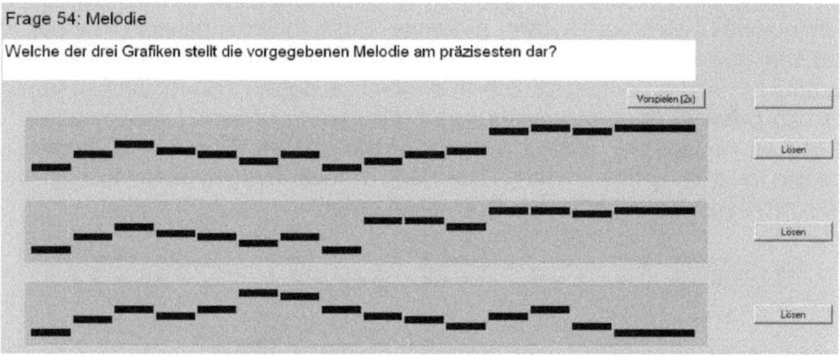

figure 5-10: transfer task in melody training of level two

The training category of rhythm, just as the above-described melody-training field, comprises listening examples of different grades of difficulty for each level, i.e. rhythms applied in level one do not reoccur in any other, higher level. The rhythms become longer and more complex with every next higher level, starting from easy rhythms of only two bars length with only two rhythmic exceptions from the ground beat for level one and progressing to rhythms of four bars length with numerous

186 For an example of a level-two graphic task in the melody-training category, see figure 5-8.

rhythmic variations for level five. 50 percent of the rhythms are in four-four measure and 50 percent in three-four measure. Level-one rhythms are either two four-four bars of crotchets ending on a minim with one crotchet replaced by two quavers or four three-four bars of crotchets ending on a dotted minim with one crotchet replaced by two quavers. Level two employs rhythms of either four four-four or three-four bars with a ground beat of crotchets ending on a minim in bar four in the case of four-four bars and on a crotchet in the case of three-four bars. One crotchet per bar is replaced by two quavers, with always two bars being identical. In this context, the first two bars and the second two bars can be identical or the outer two bars and the middle two bars or the first and the third bar and the second and the fourth bar. However, in the case of four-four bars, which end on a minim, the two crotchets in the fourth bar and its respective equal can only occur on one or two. Level-three rhythms are equally of four bars length ending on a minim with four-four bars and on a crotchet with three-four bars. In addition to the two quavers replacing one crotchet per bar, four semiquavers replace a crotchet at two random places in the rhythm and only two of the four bars are identical. Level-four rhythms consist of four four-four or three-four bars with a ground beat of quavers ending on a crotchet at the end of level four. At this stage, there are no identical bars within the rhythms. Two quavers are replaced by four semiquavers at two random places within the rhythm, two quavers are replaced by the rhythmic form of a quaver and two semiquavers, two quavers are replaced by the inverted rhythmic form of two semiquavers and a quaver and two quavers are replaced by a crotchet, all rhythmic exceptions to the ground beat occurring at random places within the rhythm with the only restriction of not forming two identical bars. Level-five rhythms, just as level-four rhythms, consist of four four-four or three-four bars with a ground beat of quavers ending on a crotchet. In addition to the above-described rhythmic forms of four semiquavers twice per rhythm, a quaver and two semiquavers once per rhythm and two semiquavers and a quaver once per rhythm, two further rhythmic variations are introduced in the context of the final level: a dotted quaver and a semiquaver replace two quavers once per rhythm and the inverted form of a semiquaver and a dotted quaver replace two further quavers of the rhythm. Figure 5-11 below displays an example of a level-five rhythm. The bars of level-five rhythms, just as those of level-four rhythms, are all different from each other.

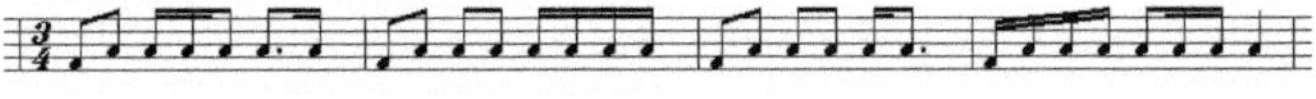

figure 5-11: level-five rhythm in ToSCA

The task of direct comparison in the context of rhythm training comprises five different kinds of answers rather than three, as in the cases of pitch and tempo training, or four, as in the melody-training category. The trainee is asked to decide whether the second rhythm is the same as the reference rhythm, whether it differs in its ending, in its beginning or its middle part or whether it differs in more than one position. Just as in the case of the above-described melody tasks, all rhythms occur in different versions in the context of this question type: one basic version, one version with an altered beginning, one version with an altered middle part and one version with an altered ending. All alterations of the basic rhythms are kept within the above-described limits of the single levels on one of bar one for a changed beginning, on four of bar one or on one of bar two in case of level-one four-four measure rhythms and on the last beat of bar two or on one of bar three in case of all other rhythms for a changed middle part and on two of the last bar in case of level-one three-four rhythms and on four of the last bar in case of all other rhythms for a changed ending. As level one mainly consists of crotchets, it does not offer many opportunities for alterations. For an altered beginning, the initial beat of the rhythm is replaced by two quavers if it is a crotchet or by a crotchet if it consists of two quavers. The altered ending introduces an additional beat to the basic-version rhythm, which already ends on three of the last bar in case of the four-four measure rhythms and on one of the last bar in case of the three-four measure rhythms. The altered-ending versions introduce either a crotchet or two quavers on the rhythm's final beat in the case of the four-four measure examples and a minim on two of the rhythm's last bar in the case of three-four measure examples, being the only rhythmic patterns introduced by this level. The altered versions of the level-two rhythms, which also consist of crotchets and quavers, exchange the respective rhythmic form of either a crotchet or two quavers with its respective counter forms of either two quavers or a crotchet at the above-described positions within the rhythm. Level three offers more opportunities for alterations already having introduced semiquavers. So the three rhythmic forms of four semiquavers, two quavers and one crotchet are interchangeable at the alteration-sensitive positions of the rhythm. Level-four alterations can take place in the form of a crotchet, two quavers, four semiquavers, two semiquavers and a crotchet or a crotchet and two semiquavers replacing the respective rhythmic form in the rhythms' positions which are due for alteration. For level five, the rhythmic forms of a dotted quaver with a semiquaver and a semiquaver with a dotted quaver are applied additionally. Especially in the context of higher levels, one could argue that the tasks dealing with three-four bars are more difficult since the rhythmic variations occur in greater density. However, this is a question of the memorising strategy applied by the trainee. If the strategy of listening to exceptions from the ground beat is applied, the four-four measure tasks are easier, but if the strategy of memorising rhythmic units is applied, the three-four measure tasks are easier. For example, the rhythmic form of four semiquavers immediately followed by the rhythmic form of two semiquavers and a quaver will not be perceived as first four semiquavers and then two extra semiquavers, which technically form a different set of rhythmic means, but, according to Gestalt theory's law of proximity, will be perceived as one entity.[187] In the context of the fifth answer option stating that the second rhythm differs in more than one position from its reference rhythm, an extra set of rhythms has been created for level one in order to avoid any coincidentally identical rhythms emerging from the basic rhythms' altered versions. The extra set of altered rhythms comprises three sets of quavers per rhythm, which can never occur in any of the other level-one rhythm versions. For levels two through five, the basic versions of the respective level's other rhythms are used for the answer option of several differences between the two rhythms to be compared, keeping the four-four measure rhythms and the three-four measures apart for obvious reasons. The program randomly chooses

187 cf. Ehrenfels 1988, Thomas 1990 and Wertheimer 1969

questions out of a selection of 120 possible tasks for level one and 108 possible tasks for levels two through five.

The recognition task in the rhythm-training category employs the rhythms' basic versions as reference rhythms and the same basic rhythms as well as their above-described altered versions, excluding the extra set of level-one rhythms, as answer options. The trainee is asked to identify the reference rhythm out of four rhythms: the basic version, the altered-beginning version, the altered-middle version and the altered-ending version. The program has a selection of 12 possible tasks per level at its disposal.

In a further question type as a part of the rhythm-training category, the trainee is asked to identify the one rhythm out of four which differs most from its reference rhythm. In this context, the rhythms' basic versions are applied as reference rhythms and their above-described altered versions are used as wrong answer options. The rhythm sought after in this kind of task stems from an extra set of altered rhythms, the rhythms of which deviate twice as much as their normally altered versions. For level one, this extra set of alterations has already been introduced above in the context of the direct-comparison tasks. All other rhythms are additionally changed by one more beat in addition to their already altered rhythmic forms, which are used as a base for the longer altered versions. This means that the normal altered-beginning version receives an additional change on two of the first bar to form the long altered-beginning version, the normal altered-middle version receives an additional change on either four of bar two, if the previous change was made on one of bar three, or vice versa, to form the long altered-middle version and the normal altered-ending version receives an additional change on either one of the last bar in the case of the three-four bars or two of the last bar in case of the four-four bars to form the long altered-ending version.[188] The program randomly poses questions out of a selection of 288 possible tasks for level one and 144 possible tasks for levels two through five.

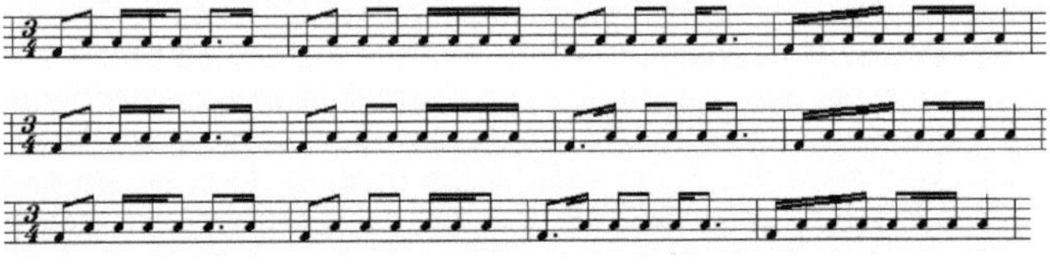

figure 5-12: level-five rhythm basic version and altered-middle versions

The transfer task in the category of rhythm training, just as the one in melody training, makes use of automatically generated graphics rather than actual pictures. The trainee is asked to match the heard reference melody with one of the graphical representations of rhythms actually occurring in the rhythm-training category of ToSCA. The rhythms' basic versions are employed as reference rhythms in this context and the graphical representations of the normal altered versions as well as of the long altered versions are used as possible wrong answers to be presented together with the matching graphical representation of the reference rhythm as a

188 For a comparison between the basic version, the normal altered-middle version and the long altered-middle version using the example of a level-five rhythm, see figure 5-10.

correct answer. Figure 5-13 below displays an example of a graphical representation of a level-three rhythm as occurring in the transfer tasks in the context of the rhythm-training category of ToSCA. The program has a selection of 108 possible tasks at its disposal for level one and 72 possible tasks for levels two through five.

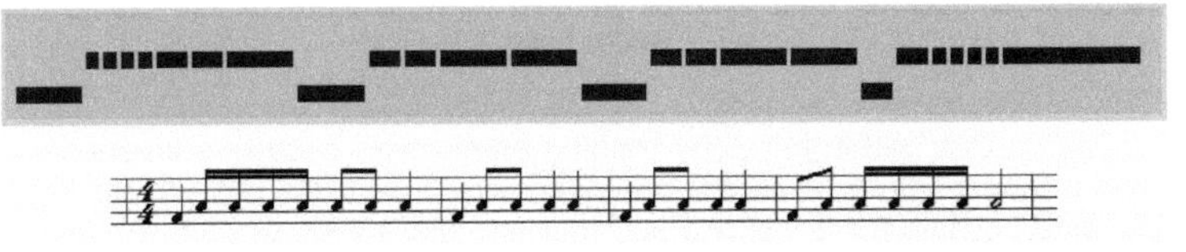

figure 5-13: example of a graphical representation of a level-three rhythm

The fifth training category within ToSCA consists of four different question types which are focused on harmony training: comparison between two harmonies, recognition of a reference harmony out of a set of three harmonies, identifying the harmonic ending out of a selection of three endings which does not lead the beginning of a cadence back to its tonic, and identifying the one harmonic movement out of three answer options which leads the reference cadence back to its tonic and thus forms a logical solution of the cadence. The basic triads employed for the comparison tasks are available in all three inversions in close position, wide position with the smallest interval being a perfect fifth and extra wide position with the smallest occurring interval being a minor tenth in all minor and major keys.[189] The trainee is to compare a reference triad with a second triad and has to decide whether the second listening example is sadder, happier or the same. For level one, only close-position triads are applied and both harmonies are played in the same inversion so, in case of two different harmonies, only the third was changed by a halftone upwards in case of a minor triad as a reference harmony and a major triad as a comparative harmony or downwards in case of a major triad as a reference harmony and a minor triad as a comparative harmony. With all existing minor and major chords matching these criteria, ToSCA can choose from 144 different questions to pose for the first level. The second level also employs close-position triads but the respective other triad to compare with the reference harmony is played in a different inversion, so that more than one tone changes for the listener. This results in 216 possible tasks for ToSCA to choose from. Level-three and level-four tasks of this question type make use of the above-introduced wide-position triads with level three applying the respective harmonies' same inversions and level four playing different inversions to compare with the reference harmony. Thus, ToSCA randomly poses questions out of a selection of 144 possible tasks for level three and 216 possible tasks for level four. Level five finally introduces the triads in extra wide position asking the trainee to compare different inversions of the harmonies in 216 possible questions.

189 See figure 5-12 for g-major in its first inversion as an example of an applied triad in close position, wide position and extra wide position.

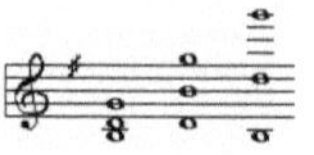

figure 5-14: close position, wide position and extra wide position for the example of a g-major triad

The recognition task within harmony training employs all occurring inversions of the minor and major triads as reference harmonies in either close position for levels one and five, wide position for levels two and four and extra wide position for level three. The different levels focus on the differentiation between varying aspects, hence the at first glance seemingly backward-moving difficulty grade after level three. Level-one and level-two tasks continue to work on the differentiation between minor and major keys, making use of all inversions of the respective other mode's key as additional wrong answer options in either close position for level one or wide position for level two. Levels three through five focus on the differentiation between the different inversion of one and the same key, which is easiest for the extra wide position with an audible difference in pitch of more than an octave trained in level three, more difficult for the harmonies in wide position with an audible pitch difference of at least a perfect fifth, which are trained in level four, and most difficult for the close-position harmonies, the outer interval of which never exceeds a major sixth and which are trained in level five. In all levels, the trainee is asked to recognise the reference harmony's twin from a set of three harmonies. The program randomly chooses questions out of a selection of 216 possible tasks for levels one and two and 72 possible tasks for levels three through five. [190]

The third question type within the category of harmony training focuses on the anticipation of cadence endings ranging from standard tonic, subdominant, dominant cadence openings to more complex cadences which are to be completed by more than one triad. The trainee is asked to identify the one triad, in case of levels one and two, or the one cadence ending, in case of levels three through five, which does not lead the respective cadence opening to a logical conclusion, from a set of three answer options. Level-one cadence openings in major consist of two triads and one four-note chord in close position: tonic, subdominant and dominant seventh, with the latter chord being an exception and all other chords occurring in the context of harmony training voiced as triads. The seventh is used in the context of level one to create a stronger dominant sound with a greater urge to resolve to the tonic. The same effect of greater tension is achieved for minor-key tasks by applying a major dominant. The program randomly picks wrong answer options with the tonic in either one of the three possible inversions in close position or resolving the preceding cadence opening to the tonic in the closest proximate wide position. The closest proximate progression to the supertonic, the mediant and the diminished triad on VII are applied as wrong cadence endings, which constitute the correct answers in this

190 The beta version of ToSCA featured a further question type between the recognition and the anticipation tasks asking the trainee to identify the one harmony out of three which differs the most from its reference harmony. However this kind of task was left out in the final version applied in the context of this study since it was found to be too ambiguous to answer in the course of beta testing.

specific question type. Level two makes use of a simple tonic, subdominant, dominant cadence opening played in wide position. The dominant in major-key tasks is played without the seventh at this stage of the training and the dominant in minor-key tasks is a minor dominant. The correct cadence endings which represent the wrong answer options are the three possible conversions of the tonic in wide position and the tonic in the close position which is closest to the preceding dominant. The next proximate subdominant, a repetition of the previously played dominant and the next proximate submediant are applied as wrong cadence endings and correct answer options. Level three employs deceptive cadence openings as reference cadences with tonic, subdominant, dominant and submediant in close position and progressions of two triads as answer options. Correct cadence endings and thus wrong answer options for level three consist of either dominant, tonic or supertonic, tonic or subdominant, tonic or mediant, tonic progressions in close position. The dominant, tonic progression occurs in three different versions: the tonic in root position, in first inversion or in second inversion and the dominant in the respective position between the preceding submediant and the final tonic. All other progressions in the context of level three occur in two different versions with the final tonic introduced from below or from above. The wrong cadence endings and thus the correct answers in this context are tonic, subdominant as well as supertonic, dominant and dominant, submediant progressions. Level-four tasks employ the same cadencial progressions for both the reference-cadence openings and the cadence endings occurring as answer options for level-three questions. All triads of level four, however, are played in wide position rather than close position. Level-five cadence openings consist of a tonic, subdominant, dominant, submediant, mediant progression in wide position. By this stage, all occurring answer options end on the respective example's tonic. The cadence endings sought after in this context are all subdominant, dominant, tonic progressions with either a missing fifth in the tonic, with the complete cadence ending in a different octave or with the tonic ending in either close or extra wide position. Other cadence endings employed as possible wrong answer options in this context are subdominant, dominant, tonic progressions with the tonic introduced from below, submediant, dominant, tonic progressions with the tonic introduced from below or from above, submediant, mediant, tonic progressions with the tonic introduced from below or from above, subdominant, mediant, tonic progressions with the tonic introduced from below or from above, submediant, diminished seventh step triad, tonic progressions with the tonic introduced from below or from above. Figure 5-15 below gives an example of a level-five cadence opening. In the context of this question type, the program randomly poses questions out of a selection of 1,296 possible tasks for levels one and two and 7,776 possible tasks for levels three through five.

The last question type within harmony training focuses on the anticipation of cadence endings just like the question type explained above. In the context of this task type, however, the trainee is asked to solve the inverted problem and to identify the one cadence ending out of a set of three answer options which leads the reference-cadence opening to a logical ending. ToSCA makes use of the same sets of cadence openings and cadence endings as answer options as explained above. However, the answer options occur in inverted roles with this question type: the correct cadence endings which lead the cadence back to its original tonic are the ones sought after here, whereas the wrong cadence endings occur in the context of wrong answer options additionally generated by the program. The program randomly issues tasks out of a set of 216 possible questions for levels one through four and 720 possible questions for level five.

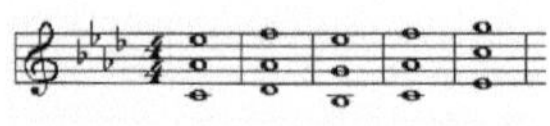

figure 5-15: cadence opening used as a reference cadence in level five

As shown in this chapter, the same question types filled with the respective training category's contents are used throughout all training fields of ToSCA. The main reason for this is to keep the phrasing of the single tasks as easy as possible in order to focus on the aspect of training and to avoid any unnecessary difficulties outside the level-specific requirements for the distinction between listening examples, the recognition of previously heard musical elements and the anticipation of endings. All listening examples applied in the context of ToSCA have been composed by the author of this dissertation according to the respective training categories' and the respective levels' specifications. In the context of training with ToSCA, it was of great importance to present previously unheard musical material and not to use already available music examples from literature in order to keep the trainees' attention focused on the tasks at hand and not on secondary thoughts such as wondering where he or she has heard the presented piece of music before. All programming work was carried out by Dr. rer. nat. Henning Sternemann.

6 Examination

6.1 Methods, Subjects and Structure of the Examination

25 subjects, henceforth called trained group, underwent an examination consisting of three phases described in detail below. 25 further subjects, henceforth called control group, took part in the first and third step of the examination leaving out the interventional phase of the experiment. All 50 test persons were students of non-linguistic subjects at German universities and none of the test persons has taken part in either instrumental or vocal education or received any other kind of training in music beyond the obligatory music education at school prior to the experiment. The trained group consisted of 11 female and 14 male subjects between 21 and 30 years of age and the control group consisted of 14 female and 11 male subjects between 20 and 33 years of age.

In the first testing phase, the subjects were surveyed on their prior experience with and education in foreign languages and on their music-consumption habits in a questionnaire and subsequently underwent a pre-intervention examination on sound discrimination and word recognition in a foreign language. The questionnaire was intended to reveal the subjects' linguistic and musical starting points at the beginning of the study and was eventually used to disclose potential relationships between certain musical habits and the performance in the music intervention described below as well as the receptivity to and the achievement in the intervention. Prior education in foreign languages was surveyed to exclude subjects with knowledge in the language to be tested and to account for possible relationships between the knowledge of certain foreign languages or the amount of foreign languages learned and the performance in the language tests. The subjects were asked to specify details about their prior linguistic education stating the languages hitherto learned, the contexts in which these languages had been acquired, namely at school, in courses, abroad, or in yet a different context to be specified, the duration of the subjects' training in the respective languages, the time elapsed since these languages were studied, and the subjects' current use of the stated languages. This part of the questionnaire was meant to reveal the subjects' past and current involvement in the process of foreign language acquisition and application as well as the diversity of languages learned and the familiarity with foreign linguistic sound patterns to be expected from the experience gathered with a certain amount of foreign languages previously learned. The same questionnaire featured a second set of questions on the subjects' preferences for music types and their average daily exposure to music. The subjects were asked to state their favourite and most consumed kind of music in order to draw possible connections between an extended exposure to either rhythm-focused music genres, such as rap music, or melody-focused music genres, such as pop music, and the subjects' performance in rhythmic and melodic tasks of the music intervention. Furthermore, it was surveyed to what extent and intensity the stated types of music are being actively listened to and passively perceived as background music. The subjects were additionally asked to specify their personal involvement in the music listened to by clapping, drumming or singing along in order to be able to hypothesise on the subjects' personal strength being more of rhythmic or more of melodic nature. In spite of all the subjects' inexperience in the learning and playing of musical instruments, certain differences in their musicality were expected. Therefore the subjects were asked to specify exactly which melody they sang and which rhythm they clapped or tapped: the main melody or the even general beat of the song, a different melody or rhythm from the song, or a self-created melody or rhythm matching the song. The survey was a combination of an open and a closed questionnaire. Most questions, such as the survey on the current use and learning of foreign languages were limited to simple yes-no answer options. However, questions on the subjects' preferred types of music and learned languages were deliberately left without pre-set answer options for several reasons. The specification of learned languages as well as the types of music listened to was left open in order to allow for the indication of possibly learned fictive languages or dialects and more specific types of music than the general main genres. Furthermore, the open questionnaire style was of great importance for the questions on music styles in order to force the subjects to state those types of music they would think of themselves and in order to prevent the effect of sudden decisions for types of music the subjects would otherwise not have stated just because of their occurrence in pre-set lists. Other closed-questionnaire type of questions included more than the above-mentioned yes-no answer options, however, always employing an even number of answer options in order to indicate a tendency and to avoid the subjects' deciding for a middle option without any statement. For the complete questionnaire, please refer to Appendix C.

The pre-intervention examination on the subjects' sound-discrimination abilities in the foreign language unknown to them was carried out via an online multiple-choice test. For details on the test's structure and characteristics, please refer to chapter 4.2.2 above.

In the second testing phase, the trained subjects underwent a non-theory based musical hearing training in the discrimination of pitch, tempo, melodies, rhythms and harmonies. The computer-based training program employed in this context is described in chapter 5.2.2 above.

The third testing phase consisted of a second language test equivalent to the above-referred-to pre-intervention examination and a self-evaluation survey on the subjects' impressions of their own achievements in both sound-discrimination tests. After two weeks of either musical hearing training in the case of the trained group or pausing in the case of the control group, both the trained subjects and the control group took part in a second sound-discrimination test of the same kind as the previously carried out pre-intervention test. To grant comparability, the second test consisted of the same questions as the first test with different words and phrases of the same level of complexity as described in chapter 4.2.2 above.

As a conclusion of the experimental phase, the subjects of both groups were asked to estimate their performances in both tests and to provide a self-evaluation on potential improvements in achievement with the second language test. This survey was carried out among the control group as well as for the trained group in order to compare to what extent the second test is subject to a familiarisation with the previously unknown language and to what extent the trained subjects' self-evaluation differs from the control groups' estimations. In differently worded questions, the subjects were asked to state which of the tests they experienced as more difficult, whether they experienced either of the tests as extremely easy or difficult, whether they managed to get used to the sounds of the previously unknown language, how quickly they were able to adapt to the new sound patterns and how they estimated their performances in both tests. For the complete survey, please refer to Appendix C.

6.2 Hypotheses

The main hypothesis of the present study focuses on the difference in performance enhancement from the first sound-discrimination test to the second for the different groups of subjects. Both the trained group and the control group were expected to improve their test performance. However, the trained group was expected to show a greater increase in both the number of correctly answered questions and the achieved total score than the control group. In addition to the total test performances, the trained group's performance in the single test-question categories on a) word order, b) words heard at specific slots of sentences, c) the identification of heard words in writing, d) the location of words in heard sentences, e) the identification of written words in acoustic form, f) the identification of words in sentences deviating in their written representations from their acoustic representations, g) the identification of written sentences in acoustic form and h) the number of words heard in sentences were expected to increase more than the control group's. For the different grades of difficulty, the difference between the single groups' increase in the number of correctly answered questions was expected to be stronger for the high-score questions than for the low-score questions, which were expected to be rather well mastered by both groups in the first sound-discrimination test already.

The hypotheses on the influence of certain training fields within the musical hearing training ToSCA on the subjects' performance improvement in the sound-discrimination tests naturally excluded the control group, which did not take part in the training with ToSCA. A high maximum score achieved in the five different training fields of pitch, tempo, melody, rhythm and harmony was expected to come along with a greater increase in both the achieved final score and the number of correct answers in the second sound-discrimination test. From the pre-study point of view, it was impossible to predict any specific correlations between the subjects' performance in single training fields of ToSCA and the score and correct-answers increase for the single question categories of the second sound-discrimination test. However, it was expected that the single training fields of ToSCA had a varying degree of influence on the single question types of the tests. In particular, rhythm and tempo as the time-oriented training categories were expected to positively influence the sound-discrimination test categories dealing with the number of words heard in a sentence, the word heard at a specific slot of a sentence, the location of a word in a sentence and the word order in a sentence. The space-oriented training categories being pitch, melody and harmony, on the other hand, were expected to show a positive effect on the question categories testing the ability to identify a written word in acoustic form, a heard word in writing, a heard sentence in writing and the word differing in the acoustic representation of a sentence from its written representation.

The influence of the subjects' musical listening and participating habits also excluded the control group for the above-stated reason. The subjects of the trained group were expected to achieve scores of varying quality within the single training fields in ToSCA depending on their daily amount of time spent on listening to music, on their taking part in the music listened to and on the kinds of music listened to. It was expected that subjects with a preference for rhythm-focused types of music would achieve higher scores in the rhythm and tempo training categories of ToSCA than other subjects, whereas subjects with a preference for melody-focused types of music would achieve higher scores in the melody and pitch training categories of ToSCA than other subjects. Furthermore it was expected that subjects with a preference for bi- or trifocal types of music would achieve higher scores in the harmony training category as well as a higher summed score than other subjects. For the subjects' achievement in the training field of melody, it was expected that subjects taking part in the music listened to by singing would achieve higher scores than those not singing, with the singing of the main voice, the singing of another voice from the music or the singing of a spontaneously invented voice matching the music being more beneficial for a high score in melody training respectively. Active participation in the music listened to by drumming or clapping along was expected to have a similar effect on the achieved score in rhythm training of ToSCA with the drumming of a rhythm occurring in the music being more beneficial for the score achieved in rhythm training than the drumming of the general beat and the spontaneous invention of a new rhythm matching the music being most beneficial. The daily time spent on actively listening to music was expected to have a positive effect on the subjects' receptivity to the training with ToSCA and thus on the score increase from one training session to the next within the above-defined fields of training for the respective types of music stated as listened to by the subjects. The number of different types of music stated as listened to by the subjects was expected to reveal information on the subjects' openness towards different types of music including the music applied in ToSCA and thus to have an effect on the maximum scores achieved for the single training categories of ToSCA. Furthermore the number of different foci of the types of music stated as listened to by the subjects was expected to have a positive effect on the maximum scores achieved as well as the score increase from one session to the next.

The influence of the subjects' prior foreign-language learning and application experience applied for both the trained and the control group. It was hypothesised that the number of languages learned at school as well as in an out-of-school context should would have a positive effect on the final score and the number of correct answers in the first test already as well as on the increase in score and the number of correct answers from the first to the second sound-discrimination test. In this context, it was expected that the number of foreign languages learned in a context out of school would be more beneficial for the achievement in the tests than the number of languages learned at school, which has the connotation of a compulsory learning activity. The time elapsed since the last foreign-language learning activity was expected to be the more beneficial for the subjects' achievement in the sound-discrimination tests the shorter it is. Both the number of foreign languages stated as currently being learned and as currently used in every-day life were hypothesised to have a positive effect on the subjects' final scores and number of correct answers as well as on the increase in score and the increase in the number of correct answers from the first to the second sound-discrimination test. Furthermore a high number of summed up foreign-language learning years was expected to have the same positive effect on the subjects' test performance.

The comparison between the subjects' self-evaluation and their actual test-performance was expected to be different for the trained group and for the control group. The control group was generally expected to evaluate their performance more hesitantly, rather making use of the middle options of "rather true" and "rather not true" than the extreme options "true" and "not true", whereas the trained group was expected to make clearer statements, choosing the extreme options over the middle ones. The trained group was expected to evaluate their performance in the second test as clearly better than in the first test, whereas the control group was expected to state that the second test was experienced as vaguely less difficult. It was expected that both groups experience the first sound-discrimination test as more difficult than the second one and that the first test is more likely to be labelled as "extremely difficult" than the second one. Subjects stating that they were able to immediately get used to the sound of the new language were expected to achieve a high score with a large number of correct answers in the first test already, whereas subjects stating that they had been able to gradually get used to the sound of the new language in the course of the two tests were expected to achieve a high increase in their score and their number of correct answers from the first to the second sound-discrimination test. In contrast, subjects stating that they had not been able to get used to the sound of the new language at all were expected to finish both tests with relatively low scores and a relatively low number of correct answers. For those statements of the self-evaluation survey which directly compare the first sound-discrimination test with the second one, the subjects of both groups are expected to make realistic estimations on their performance, again with the control group being more hesitant in their statements than the trained group.

6.3 Results

6.3.1 Influence of ToSCA on the Subjects' Performance in the Sound-Discrimination Tests

The post-intervention sound-discrimination test resulted in a statistically significant improvement in the number of correct answers given by the subjects of the trained group as opposed to their results on the pre-intervention test. Even though the control group was able to answer more questions correctly in the post-intervention test as well, the mean difference in their results remained without statistical significance. Both groups were able to improve their mean final scores in the second test, however, without any statistically significant difference. The difference between the mean score increase of the trained group and that of the control group, just as the difference between the mean increase in the number of correct answers given by the trained group and that of the control group, failed to prove statistically significant, an effect which was possibly caused by an insufficient number of subjects.

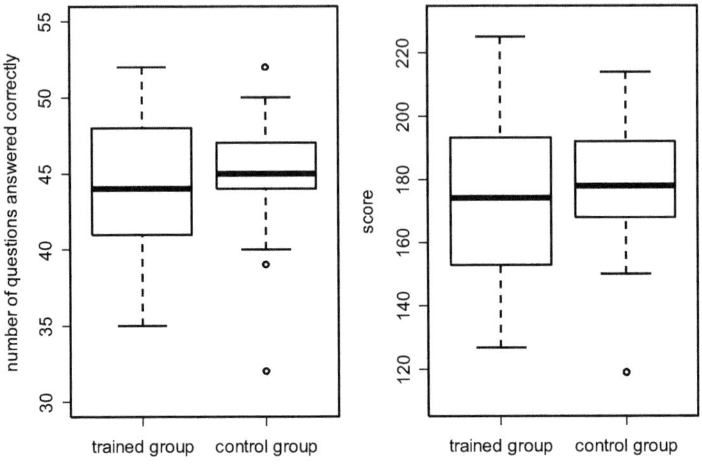

figure 6-16: summary of the results achieved in the first sound-discrimination test

The initial situation of the subjects' sound-discrimination abilities as tested in the pre-intervention examination in the course of the first testing phase proved to be uneven for the two groups with a better result for the control group. As the boxplots in figure 6.16 above reveal, the number of correct answers given in the first test shows a smaller interquartile range for the control group than it does for the trained group with a median of 45 answers for the control group and 44 answers for the trained group. The results of the control group lie between 40 and 50 correct answers neglecting the three values indicated as outliers located at 32, 39 and 52 answers as opposed to the trained group's results ranging from 35 to 52 correct answers. The interquartile range for the trained group amounts to 7, ranging from 41 to 48, whereas that of the control group amounts to 3, only ranging from 44 to 47. As shown in figure 6.16 above, the comparison of the scores achieved in the first sound-discrimination test reveals a similar situation, with the control group's results showing a smaller interquartile range than the trained group's. Again not taking the single outlier of 119 points within the control group into account, the trained group's results range from 127 to 225 as opposed to the control group's results, which range from 150 to 214. The trained group's interquartile range amounts to 40, ranging from 153 to 193, with a median of 174, in contrast to an interquartile range of 24, ranging from 168 to 192, with a median of 178, for the control group. For this reason, the following observations will focus on the mean of the subjects' personal improvement in the number of correct answers and in the scores achieved more strongly than on the direct comparison of total scores and numbers of correct answers.[191]

191 For a comprehensive overview of all test results, refer to Appendix A.1.

The comparison of the mean score increase and the mean increase in the number of correct answers from the first to the second sound-discrimination test between the trained group and the control group resulted in a positive difference for both groups with a slightly stronger difference for the trained group. The trained group was able to achieve a total score being a mean of 6.84 points higher in the second sound-discrimination test than in the first and succeeded in raising their number of correct answers by a mean of 1.8. The control group achieved a mean score rise of 5.6 points and a mean increase in the number of correct answers of 1.32.[192]

When comparing the detailed results of the single question categories employed in the course of the sound-discrimination tests, it can be observed that the trained group was able to achieve a better mean score increase as well as a higher mean increase in the number of correct answers than the control group for questions on the amount of words in a sentence, the location of a word in a sentence and the identification of a written word in acoustic form. The trained group achieved a mean score increase of 2.96 points and a mean increase in the number of correct answers of 1.24, as opposed to a mean score increase of 2.28 points and a mean increase in the number of correct answers of 0.84 achieved by the control group for questions on the number of words in a sentence. For questions on the location of a word in a sentence, the trained group was able to reach a mean 3.24-point score raise and a mean increase in the number of correct answers by 0.52, as opposed to a 0.28-point score raise and a mean increase in the number of correct answers of 0.08 achieved by the control group. Furthermore, the trained group was able to increase the score for questions on the identification of a written word in acoustic form by a mean of 0.48 points and the number of correct answers by a mean of 0.16 in contrast to the control group, which experienced a negative trend for both the score lowered by a mean of 0.92 points and the number of correctly answered questions lowered by a mean of 0.16.

The test-question categories dealing with the identification of a heard word in written form and the identification of the word differing in the written representation of a sentence from its acoustic representation experienced a mean loss in score as well as in the number of correct answers for both the trained and the control group. The trained group, however, experienced smaller losses than the control group. The mean score loss for questions on the identification of a heard word in written form amounts to 1.56 points for the trained group and 2.72 points for the control group. The mean difference between the number of correct answers given for this category in the second and the first sound-discrimination tests amounts to -0.12 for the trained group and -0.4 for the control group. The largest score decline within a question category is to be observed for questions on the identification of the word differing in its written representation from its acoustic representation, for which the trained group experienced a mean decline of 3.36 points and the control group of 4.2 points. The number of questions answered correctly within this category decreased by 0.56 in the case of the trained group and by 0.68 in the case of the control group.

The control group was able to achieve a better mean increase in both score and the number of correct answers for questions on the word heard at a specific slot of a

192 For a detailed overview of all data on the difference in score and the number of correct answers, refer to table 6-b below.

sentence and questions on the identification of a written sentence in acoustic form. The trained group was able to obtain a mean score raise of 2.28 points for questions on the word heard at a specific slot of a sentence as opposed to a mean score raise of 4 points achieved by the control group. The same question category resulted in an increase in the number of correct answers of 0.24 for the trained group and of 0.52 by the control group. For questions on the identification of a written sentence in acoustic form, the trained group obtained a mean raise in score of 3.32 points and a mean raise in the number of correct answers of 0.52, in contrast to a mean score raise of 4.44 points and a mean raise in the number of correct answers of 0.64 achieved by the control group.

The score and number of correct answers for questions on the order of words in a sentence exhibited opposing trends for the trained group and the control group. Whereas the control group was able to achieve a mean raise in score of 3.64 points and number of correct answers of 0.48, the trained group experienced a mean score decline of 0.52 points and a decrease of the number of correct answers of 0.2.

When comparing the trained group's and the control group's increase in correct answers within the different grades of difficulty of the sound-discrimination tests, the lower four grades of difficulty showed a positive difference for both groups, with the trained group achieving larger differences than the control group. The trained group was able to achieve a mean increase in correct answers of 0.4 for grade-one questions, 0.56 for grade-two questions, 0.2 for grade-three questions and 0.8 for grade-four questions as opposed to a mean increase in correct answers of 0.32 for grade-one questions, 0.28 for grade-two questions, 0.12 for grade-three questions and 0.32 for grade-four questions achieved by the control group. Furthermore, both groups were able to obtain a higher mean number of correct answers within the upper two grades of difficulty, with the control group achieving larger differences than the trained group. The trained group achieved a mean increase of 0.16 as opposed to a mean increase of 0.28 obtained by the control group for grade-eight questions. The number of correct answers for questions with the highest grade of difficulty rose by 0.6 for the trained group and by 0.64 for the control group. Both groups experienced a decrease in the number of correct answers given for questions with a grade-seven difficulty. The mean decrease amounts to 0.76 for the trained group and 0.4 for the control group. The number of correct answers given for questions with a grade-five and grade-six level of difficulty reveal opposing trends for the two groups, with a positive difference for grade-six questions in favour of the trained group and a positive difference for grade-five questions in favour of the control group. Within the fifth level of difficulty, the trained group saw a mean decrease in the number of correct answers of 0.4, whereas the control group managed to achieve a mean increase of 0.08. Within the sixth level of difficulty, the trained group obtained a mean increase in the number of correct answers of 0.36, whereas the control group suffered a mean decrease of 0.24.

	increase in	mean of trained group	mean of control group	diff. [193]	p-value	t-value	conf. int.[194]
total tests	No. of correct answers	1.80	1.32	0.48	0.33	-0.45	-∞, 1.29
	score	6.84	5.60	1.24	0.42	-0.19	-∞, 9.55
category 1	No. of correct answers	1.24	0.84	0.4	0.23	-0.75	-∞, 0.50
	score	2.96	2.28	0.68	0.40	-0.26	-∞, 3.63
category 2	No. of correct answers	0.24	0.52	-0.28	0.76	0.71	-∞, 0.94
	score	2.28	4.00	-1.72	0.74	0.65	-∞, 6.16
category 3	No. of correct answers	-0.12	-0.40	0.28	0.14	-1.10	-∞, 0.15
	score	-1.56	-2.72	1.16	0.23	-0.73	-∞, 1.49
category 4	No. of correct answers	0.52	0.08	0.44	0.12	-1.19	-∞, 0.18
	score	3.24	0.28	2.96	0.12	-1.21	-∞, 1.15
category 5	No. of correct answers	0.16	-0.16	0.32	0.18	-0.92	-∞, 0.26
	score	0.48	-0.92	1.4	0.24	-0.72	-∞, 1.86
category 6	No. of correct answers	-0.20	0.48	-0.68	0.96	1.72	-∞, 1.34
	score	-0.52	3.64	-4.16	0.94	1.58	-∞, 8.58
category 7	No. of correct answers	-0.56	-0.68	0.12	0.34	-0.43	-∞, 0.35
	score	-3.36	-4.20	0.84	0.27	-0.62	-∞, 1.44
category 8	No. of correct answers	0.52	0.64	-0.12	0.65	0.40	-∞, 0.62
	score	3.32	4.44	-1.12	0.79	0.80	-∞, 3.45
difficulty grade 1	No. of correct answers	0.40	0.32	0.08	0.36	-0.35	-∞, 0.30
difficulty grade 2	No. of correct answers	0.56	0.28	0.28	0.11	-1.23	-∞, 0.10
difficulty grade 3	No. of correct answers	0.20	0.12	0.08	0.35	-0.39	-∞, 0.26
difficulty grade 4	No. of correct answers	0.80	0.32	0.48	0.06	-1.58	-∞, 0.03
difficulty grade 5	No. of correct answers	-0.40	0.08	-0.48	0.91	1.33	-∞, 1.08
difficulty grade 6	No. of correct answers	0.36	-0.24	0.6	0.09	-1.39	-∞, 0.13
difficulty grade 7	No. of correct answers	-0.76	-0.40	-0.36	0.82	0.92	-∞, 1.02
difficulty grade 8	No. of correct answers	0.16	0.28	-0.12	0.64	0.35	-∞, 0.69

193 difference between the mean improvement achieved by the trained group and the mean improvement achieved by the control group

194 confidence interval

difficulty grade 9	No. of correct answers	0.60	0.64	-0.04	0.54	0.11	-∞, 0.66

table 6-b: mean differences in scores achieved and the number of correct answers given in the second and the first sound-discrimination test

A two-sided One Sample t-test on the null hypothesis of the true mean equalling zero was carried out for the score increase of all subjects, the increase in the number of correct answers given by all subjects, the score increase within the control group, the increase in the number of correct answers given by the control group, the score increase within the trained group and the increase in the number of correct answers given by the trained group. In this context, the test statistic T is given by

$$T = \sqrt{n}\frac{\overline{X}}{S} \qquad (6.1)$$

the square root of the number of subjects n multiplied with the mean $\overline{X}$ of the data divided by the standard deviation S. Finally, T is compared with the corresponding quantiles of a t distribution using a significance level of $\alpha = 0.05$ so that the null hypothesis can be rejected in case of the p-value remaining smaller than α.

As displayed in table 6-c below, the mean increase in the number of correct answers for the whole group was found to be highly significant with a p-value of 0.005. When looking at the results of the separate groups, the increase in the number of correct answers also proved statistically significant for the trained group with a p-value of 0.02, whereas only a small tendency could be seen for the control group, with a p-value rounded down to 0.10. The score increase achieved by the complete group showed a trend towards the rejection of the null hypothesis with a p-value of 0.06, whereas none of the results achieved by the single groups separately revealed any statistical significance, with p-values of 0.15 for the trained group and 0.22 for the control group.

		mean	p-value	t-value	conf. int.
all	score increase	6.22	0.06	-1.95	-12.62 - 0.18
	increase in number of correct answers	1.56	0.005	-2.98	-2.61 - -0.51
trained group	score increase	6.84	0.15	-1.48	-16.38 - 2.70
	increase in number of correct answers	1.8	0.02	-2.50	-3.28 - -0.32
control group	score increase	5.6	0.22	-1.25	-14.84 - 3.64
	increase in number of correct answers	1.32	0.10	-1.71	-2.92 - 0.28

table 6-c: mean increase in score and in the number of correct answers for all subjects and for the two groups separately

A one-sided Welch Two Sample t-test on the null hypothesis of the trained group achieving larger or equally increased values than the control group in the second sound-discrimination test compared to the first one revealed no statistically significant differences. In this context, the mean values $\overline{X}_c$ achieved by the control group minus the mean values $\overline{X}_t$ achieved by the trained group were divided by the pooled standard deviations of the two groups' values, i.e. the square root of the sum of (i) the control group's estimated variance $S^2{}_{X_c}$ divided by the number of subjects, n=25, in this group and (ii) the trained group's estimated variance $S^2{}_{X_t}$ divided by the number of subjects, m=25, in this group. Therefore the test statistic T is given by

$$T = \frac{\overline{X_c} - \overline{X_t}}{\sqrt{\frac{S^2{}_{Xc}}{n} + \frac{S^2{}_{Xt}}{m}}}. \qquad (6.2)$$

The test statistic T is finally compared with the corresponding quantile of a t distribution using a significance level of $\alpha = 0.05$ so that the null hypothesis can be rejected in case of the p-value remaining smaller than α. A trend towards a rejection of the null hypothesis could be seen especially for the increase in the number of two-point, four-point and six-point questions with p-values of 0.11, 0.06 and 0.09 respectively and, to a smaller extent, for the increase in the number of correct answers within question categories three through five dealing with the identification of a heard word in written form, the location of a word in a sentence and the identification of a written word in acoustic form with p-values of 0.14, 0.12 and 0.18 respectively. Furthermore, the same tendency became apparent with a p-value of 0.12 for the score increase within the question category testing the subjects' ability to locate a word in a sentence.

Furthermore, a stepwise regression[195] according to Akaike's Information Criterion[196] was carried out in order to examine the potential influence of specific training categories within ToSCA on the subjects' improvement within the single question categories of the sound-discrimination tests. In particular, the dependency of the difference in score and in the number of correct answers on the maximum scores achieved in the five ToSCA training categories of pitch, tempo, melody, rhythm and harmony and the percentage of questions answered correctly for each of the training categories was tested for the final sound-discrimination test results as well as, separately, for the eight question categories described in detail in chapter 4.2.2 above. This examination procedure revealed a statistically significant dependency of both the increase in score and in the number of correct answers given for questions on the number of words in a sentence on the maximum score achieved in the tempo training category of ToSCA. Assuming a linear context, the difference between the numbers of correct answers in the first and in the second sound-discrimination test will rise by 1, if the maximum score achieved during tempo training with ToSCA is higher by 0.08 points; and the difference between the final scores achieved in test one and in test two will rise by 1, if the maximum score achieved during tempo training is higher by 0.35 points, with a p-value of 0.02 for the increase in the number of correct answers and a p-value of 0.04 for the score

195 For details on the principle of stepwise regression, please refer to Fox (2002).

196 For details on Akaike's Information Criterion, please refer to Venables and Ripley (2002).

increase. The second question type of the sound-discrimination tests, which deals with the identification of the word heard at a certain slot within the sentence, showed a tendency to depend on the percentage of correct answers given in the melody-training category of ToSCA, in case of the increase in correct answers given in the test and on the maximum score achieved in the rhythm-training category of ToSCA in case of the test-score increase. Again assuming a linear context, the difference between the numbers of correct answers given in test one and in test two will rise by 1, if the percentage of melody questions answered correctly is higher by 0.05, and the difference between the final scores achieved will rise by 1, if the maximum score is higher by 0.33 points. The p-values of 0.09 for the influence on the score increase and rounded-down 0.05 for the increase in the number of correct answers, however, only reveal a tendency rather than a statistical significance. The third sound-discrimination test question category dealing with the identification of a heard word in writing did not reveal any dependencies on the tested explanatory variables. The fourth category, consisting of questions on the location of a word in a sentence, however, was found to depend on a high number of factors. Whereas the percentage of correctly answered pitch questions, the percentage of correctly answered melody questions and the maximum score achieved during tempo training appear as explanatory variables in negative correlation, the percentage of correctly answered rhythm questions, the maximum score achieved within pitch training and the maximum score achieved within harmony training were issued as explanatory variables in positive correlation with the difference between the numbers of correct answers in test one and test two. Still assuming a linear context, a 1 percent raised percentage of pitch questions answered correctly entails a by 0.33 lowered number of correct answers at an extremely high level of significance with a p-value of 0.0006. A 1 percent raised percentage of melody questions answered correctly as well as a 1 point raised maximum score achieved during tempo training were revealed to lower the number of correct answers given in this question category by 0.06 with a p-value of 0.13 and thus no statistical significance in the case of the melody-training category and a p-value of 0.04 and thus within the range of statistical significance in the case of the tempo-training category. The dependency of the difference between the numbers of correct answers given within this category in tests one and two on the positively correlated explanatory variables all proved to be statistically significant, with the percentage of rhythm questions answered correctly during the training with ToSCA showing the largest augmentation effect of 0.15 at a high level of statistical significance with a p-value of 0.009. The maximum score achieved within pitch training showed an augmentation effect of 0.11 points and the maximum score achieved within harmony training of 0.06 points, both with a p-value of 0.02. The difference between the scores achieved in tests one and two within the same category was issued together with the maximum score achieved within rhythm training as positively correlated explanatory variables and the percentage of pitch questions answered correctly as a negatively correlated explanatory variable. In a linear context, this means a decrease of 0.92 points for questions on the location of a word in a sentence, with every further percent added to the percentage of pitch questions answered correctly. This context proved statistically significant with a p-value of 0.01. The maximum score achieved during rhythm training with ToSCA as the positively correlated explanatory variable in this context revealed a tendency to raise the score by 0.4 points per further point in the maximum rhythm score with a p-value of 0.08. The fifth question category within the sound-discrimination tests, dealing with questions on the identification of a written word in acoustic form, was found to only show a trend towards a dependency of the number of correctly answered questions on the maximum score achieved during melody training as an explanatory variable with a slightly negative correlation. 1 point of the maximum score achieved in melody training with ToSCA tends to result in a second sound-discrimination test result decreased by 0.04 correct answers. The score difference within the same test-question category appears to be positively dependent on the maximum pitch score and negatively dependent on the maximum tempo score. Whereas the maximum pitch score shown to increase the test-score within the present category by 0.18 points did not prove statistically significant with a p-value of 0.19, the maximum tempo score appears to decrease the test-score of the fifth category by 0.29 points, revealing statistical significance with a p-value of 0.04. The sixth test-question category, consisting of questions on the word order in a sentence, did not reveal any explanatory variables at all for the difference in the numbers of correct answers given in tests one and two and only shared the percentage of pitch questions answered correctly as a statistically insignificant, negatively correlated explanatory variable of the score increase with a p-value of 0.17. Each further percent in the percentage of pitch questions answered correctly appears to decrease the score for word-order questions in the second sound-discrimination test by 0.45 points. The seventh test-question category, dealing with questions on the identification of the word differing in the written representation of a sentence from its acoustic representation, did not prove to be dependent on any of the tested factors. The eighth question category, with questions on the identification of a written sentence in acoustic form, was found to be dependent on one positively and one negatively correlated variable. The percentage of rhythm questions answered correctly appears to raise the score within this category by 0.29 points with every further percent, whereas the maximum score achieved during tempo training with ToSCA seems to decrease the score by 0.12 points for every further point. However, the positively correlated explanatory variable only proved a trend towards the rejection of the null hypothesis with a p-value of 0.08, whereas the p-value of 0.17 could not prove the negatively correlated explanatory variable statistically significant. Table 6-d below represents a summary of the above-described phenomena, with the first value within a field indicating the coefficient for linear dependency and the second one representing the p-value. The test-question categories which proved to be independent of any of the tested variables were left out in the overview as well as the tested variables which failed to prove explanatory for any of the test items.

		number of correct answers	score	number of correct answers	score	number of correct answers	score	number of correct answers	score	score	score
		category 1		category 2		category 4		category 5		cat. 6	cat. 8
questions answered	pitch					-0.33 0.0006	-0.92 0.01			-0.45 0.17	
	melody			0.05 0.09		-0.06 0.13					
	rhythm					0.15 0.009			0.18 0.19		0.29 0.08

maximum pitch score					0.11 0.02		-0.04 0.09	-0.29 0.04		
maximum tempo score	0.08 0.02	0.35 0.04			-0.06 0.04					-0.12 0.17
maximum rhythm score				0.33 0.09		0.40 0.08				
maximum harmony score					0.06 0.02					

table 6-d: overview of the sound-discrimination test results shown to be dependent on one or more training categories of ToSCA after the execution of a stepwise regression according to Akaike's Information Criterion. First value: coefficient for linear dependency. Second value: p-value.

6.3.2 Influence of the Subjects' Previous Language-Learning Experience on Their Test Performance

A stepwise regression according to Akaike's Information Criterion was carried out in order to test potentially explanatory variables for the subjects' performance in the sound-discrimination test. In this context, a) the total number of languages learned at school, b) the total number of languages learned in a voluntary, out-of-school context, c) the years elapsed since the last language-learning activity, d) the number of languages currently being learned, e) the number of languages currently used in daily life and f) the summed up language-learning years[197] were tested as potentially explanatory variables for the performance in the first sound-discrimination test and the increase in score and in the number of correct answers from the first to the second test.

Neither the total number of questions answered correctly nor the total score achieved in the first sound-discrimination test proved to be dependent on any of the tested factors.

For the difference between the total scores achieved in test one and test two and the numbers of questions answered correctly in test one and test two, the number of foreign languages currently used in daily life appeared as a single explanatory variable. Assuming a linear context, the final score achieved in test two will rise by 10.62 points for every further language currently used in daily life. This connection proved statistically significant with a p-value of 0.02. The number of questions answered correctly was found to rise by 1.21 for every further language currently used, however without any statistical significance at a p-value of 0.12.

In the testing of the single question categories of the sound-discrimination test, no explanatory variables were found for the first and the fourth category, consisting of questions on the number of words in a sentence and the location of a word in a sentence.

197 Mathematical value, which indicates the summed up numbers of years spent on learning single languages, some of which may de facto have been learned simultaneously.

The second category, containing questions on the word heard at a specific slot of a sentence, was found to be positively correlated with the number of languages currently used in daily life and negatively correlated with the number of languages learned in a voluntary context. For each further language currently used, the score increases by 3.28 points and the number of correct answers by 0.55 points within category two of the second sound-discrimination test. The p-values of rounded-down 0.05 and 0.09, however, merely indicate a trend rather than a statistical significance. Each further language learned in a voluntary context was found to decrease the score by 3.95 points and the number of questions by 0.59 within this question category. The negatively correlated explanatory variables, in contrast to the positively correlated ones, revealed statistically significant results with rounded-up p-values of 0.05.

The third category of test questions on the identification of a heard word in writing appears to be dependent on the number of foreign languages learned at school. The number of correct answers is shown to increase by 0.74 and the score by 8.49 points for each further language learned. Both results reveal a high level of statistical significance with p-values of 0.002 for the increase in the number of correct answers and 0.0008 for the score increase. The number of foreign languages learned in a voluntary context also proved to be an explanatory variable for the subjects' performance within this category. The number of correct answers shows a tendency to rise by 0.31 with a p-value of 0.09 and the score proved to rise by 4.43 points with a p-value of 0.02. The summed up language-learning years is included as an additional explanatory variable for the score increase, raising the score by 0.18 points for each further year of language learning. This additional factor also proved statistically significant with a p-value of rounded-up 0.05.

The fifth test-question category, dealing with questions on the identification of a written word in acoustic form, was only issued in context with the number of languages currently learned as a single positively correlated explanatory variable for the score increase. Without any statistical significance and with a p-value of 0.12, the category-five score seems to increase by 2.73 points for each further language currently being learned.

In the sixth test-question category, consisting of questions on the word order in a sentence, the increase in score appeared to have one negatively and one positively correlated explanatory variable, whereas the increase in the number of correct answers did not prove to be dependent on any of the tested factors. The score achieved in the sixth category within the second sound-discrimination test appears to increase by 4.57 points for every further language currently used in daily life, whereas the summed up language-learning time appears as a negatively correlated explanatory variable lowering the score by 0.27 points for every further year of language learning. Whereas the positively correlated explanatory variable proved statistically significant with a p-value of 0.04, the negatively correlated explanatory variable showed a rather vague dependency at a p-value of 0.17.

The seventh test-question category of the sound-discrimination tests was only issued in context with negatively correlated explanatory variables, all three of which revealed statistical significance. The number of languages learned in a voluntary context appeared as the strongest negatively correlated explanatory variable lowering the category-seven number of correct answers given in the second test by 0.52 and causing a score decrease of 2.89 points for each further language learned in a voluntary context. The score decrease was found to be of high statistical significance with a p-value of 0.004 and the decrease in the number of correct answers proved statistically significant as well with a p-value of 0.01. The time elapsed since the subjects' last language learning activity proved a highly significant explanatory variable with a p-value of 0.003 for both the score and the number of correct answers in the seventh test-question category. For each further year elapsed since the subjects' last language-learning activity, the score was shown to decrease by 0.48 points and the number of correct answers by 0.1. The third and last negatively correlated explanatory variable for the seventh test-question category proved to be the subjects' summed up language-learning time with p-values of 0.04, and thus statistical significance. The score appeared as decreased by 0.17 points and the number of correct answers by 0.04 for each further year of language learning.

The increase in the number of correct answers for category-eight questions on the identification of a written sentence in acoustic form only appeared with the number of languages currently used in daily life as a single and not significant explanatory variable raising the number of correct answers by 0.36 for each further language currently used. The score increase achieved within the same category, however, proved to have two positively correlated explanatory variables. The time elapsed since the subjects' last language-learning activity seems to increase the category-eight score by 0.27 points for every further year, however failing to prove significant with a p-value of 0.12. The number of languages currently used, on the other hand, appears to have a greater effect, raising the score within category eight by 2.31 points for each further language currently used, this time presenting a statistically significant result with a p-value of 0.03.

For the increase in the number of correct answers given within the range of the nine grades of difficulty in the sound-discrimination tests, no explanatory variables at all were found for the lower grades of difficulty from one to five with an exception of grade-two questions. The only statistically significant explanatory variable was found for grade-seven questions, which appear to decrease in the number of correct answers by 0.11 for every further year elapsed since the subjects' last language-learning activity. Grade-eight questions, like the lower grades of difficulty, failed to prove influenced by any of the tested factors.

The number of questions answered correctly at the second grade of difficulty showed a trend to decrease by 0.32 for each further language currently used in daily life at a p-value of 0.06.

The number of questions answered correctly within difficulty grades six and nine were shown to have only positively correlated explanatory variables. The number of correct answers at the sixth grade of difficulty revealed a tendency to increase by 0.68 for every further language currently being learned. The p-value of 0.06, however, only expresses a trend rather than a significant difference. The number of difficulty-grade-nine questions answered correctly seems to increase by 0.09 for each further year elapsed since the subjects' last language-learning activity and by 0.46 for each further language currently used in daily life. The p-values of rounded-down 0.05 for the time elapsed since the subjects' last language learning and rounded-up 0.10 for the number of languages currently used can only be seen as trend indicators.

Table 6-e below represents an overview of the results gained in the course of the above-described stepwise regression on the dependency of the subjects' performance and performance improvement in the second sound-discrimination test on their previous language-learning experience. The first value in a field indicates the degree of influence and the second represents the p-value. Sound-discrimination test elements which failed to prove dependent on any of the tested factors were left out in the overview.

		increase in	total number of FLs[198] learned at school	total number of FLs learned in a voluntary context	time elapsed since last FL-learning activity	number of FLs currently learned	number of FLs currently used	summed up FL-learning years
total test		number of correct answers					1.21 0.12	
total test		score					10.62 0.02	
category	2	number of correct answers		-0.59 0.05			0.55 0.05	
category	2	score		-3.95 0.05			3.28 0.09	
category	3	number of correct answers	0.74 0.002	0.31 0.09				
category	3	score	8.49 0.0008	4.43 0.02				0.18 0.05
category	5	score				2.73 0.12		
category	6	score					4.57 0.04	-0.27 0.17
category	7	number of correct answers		-0.52 0.01	-0.10 0.003			-0.04 0.04
category	7	score		-2.89 0.004	-0.48 0.003			-0.17 0.04
category	8	number of correct answers					0.36 0.11	
category	8	score			0.27 0.12		2.31 0.03	
grade of difficulty	2	number of correct answers					-0.32 0.06	
grade of difficulty	6	number of correct answers				0.68 0.08		
grade of difficulty	7	number of correct answers			-0.11 0.02			
grade of difficulty	9	number of correct answers			0.09 0.05		0.46 0.10	

198 FL = foreign language

table 6-e: summary of the influence of the subjects' previous language-learning experience on their performance in the sound-discrimination tests. First value: gradient in the assumed linear context. Second value: p-value.

6.3.3 Dependency of the Subjects' Receptivity to Aural Training with ToSCA on Their Musical Habits

In order to test the dependency of the subjects' receptivity to and performance in the five training categories of the aural training program ToSCA on their musical habits and preferences, a stepwise regression according to Akaike's Information Criterion was executed. In this context, a) the total number of different types of music stated as listened to by the subjects, b) the subjects' participation in the music listened to, c) the kind of voice sung when singing along to the music, d) the kind of rhythm clapped or drummed when drumming along to the music, e) the amount of different foci for the types of music stated as listened to, f) the number of melody-focused types of music stated as listened to, g) the number of rhythm-focused types of music stated as listened to, h) the number of harmony-focused types of music stated as listened to, i) the number of bi- or tri-focal types of music stated as listened to, j) the number of different musical foci occurring in the types of music stated as frequently listened to, k) the focus of the type of music stated as most listened to, l) the time spent on listening to the type of music stated as most listened to, m) the time spent on listening to other types of music stated as frequently listened to, n) the frequency of the subjects' exposure to live music and o) the subjects' self evaluation on their musical taste and development[199] were tested as potentially explanatory variables for the subjects' mean improvement from one ToSCA training session to the next for the total training and within the single training categories of pitch, tempo, melody, rhythm and harmony, the percentage of questions answered correctly for the total training and for the single training categories and the maximum scores achieved in the five categories of ToSCA.

The mean score increase for the pitch category of ToSCA was found to be positively dependent on the number of music types stated as listened to with the mean score increase rising by 0.37 points for each further type of music when assuming a linear context. This dependency proved highly significant with a p-value of 0.007. Furthermore, the kind of voice sung along to the music most listened to was revealed as an explanatory variable for the mean score increase within this category. For the lack of participation in the music by singing, the mean score was found to increase by 0.69 points, for the singing of a newly invented voice matching the music, the mean score increase rose by 0.51 points, whereas a negative dependency was shown for the singing of a melody from the music other than the main voice with a decrease of the mean score progression by 0.38 points. Neither of the singing-participation variables proved statistically significant.

The mean score increase in tempo training showed a trend towards dependency on the amount of different foci of the types of music stated as listened

199 For a complete overview of the statements the subjects were confronted with in the course of the pre-examination self-evaluation as a part of the first survey, please refer to appendix C.1.

to. Assuming a linear context, a 0.31-point raise could be shown for each further focus at a p-value of 0.07.

The mean score increase for the melody-training category of ToSCA was found to be dependent on the number of melody-focused types of music stated as listened to, the focus of the music most listened to, the participation in the music by drumming or clapping along and the time spent on actively listening to the music stated as most listened to. Every further melody-focused type of music stated as listened to proved to coincide with a mean score increase in melody training raised by 0.37 points revealing statistical significance with a p-value of 0.03. The type of music most listened to being a bi- or trifocal kind of music, on the other hand, proved a negatively correlated explanatory variable for this training category, with the mean score progression decreasing by 1.27 points at a p-value of 0.04. The participation in the music most listened to by clapping or drumming along proved most strongly dependent in the case of the drumming of newly invented rhythms matching the music, with an increase of the mean score progression by 1.37 points in a linear context, revealing statistical significance with a p-value of 0.01. The drumming along of a different rhythm occurring in the music appeared positively dependent on the mean score progression, revealing a mean score increase of 0.39 points, while the lack of participation in the music by drumming along coincided with a score increase of 0.86 points, however without any statistical significance. The time spent on actively listening to the type of music stated as most listened to appears in a negative dependency in context with the mean score progression, coinciding with a decrease of 0.35 points for every further hour spent on listening to the type of music stated as most listened to per day.

The mean score increase in the rhythm-training category of ToSCA proved most strongly dependent on the number of harmony-focused types of music stated as listened to, coinciding with a rise of the mean score progression by 1.10 points for every further type of harmony-focused music stated as listened to and on the drumming along of a rhythm occurring in the music other than the main beat to the music most listened to coinciding with an increase of the mean score progression by 1.65 points. Both explanatory variables proved statistically significant, with a p-value of 0.04 for the number of harmony-focused types of music listened to and a p-value of 0.009 for the drumming along of a rhythm occurring in the music other than the main beat to the music most listened to. The drumming along of a self-invented rhythm was stated as a negatively correlated explanatory variable coinciding with a decrease of the mean score progression in rhythm training by 0.17 points and the lack of participation in the music by drumming or clapping along appeared as a positively correlated explanatory variable coinciding with an increase of the mean score progression by 0.02 points, still assuming a linear context. Neither of these variables, however, revealed any statistical significance or even a trend, with extremely high p-values of 0.69 and 0.97. The number of different foci of the types of music stated as listened to was found to be another negatively correlated explanatory variable for the mean score increase in rhythm training coinciding with a decrease of 0.34 points for every further focus occurring within the types of music listened to.

The mean score increase in harmony training proved to be most strongly dependent on the participation in the music stated as most listened to by singing. The singing along of a voice occurring in the music other than the main voice coincided with an increase of the mean score progression in harmony training of 1.5 points and the singing of a self-invented voice matching the music corresponded with a rise of the mean score increase of 2.11 points. Both explanatory variables proved highly statistically significant with p-values of 0.006 and 0.007. The lack of participation in the music most listened to by singing, however, also proved a positive dependency on the mean score progression increasing by 1.20 points with a p-value of 0.03 and thus revealing statistical significance. Furthermore, the number of melody-focused types of music showed a trend towards a positive dependency on the mean score increase rising by 0.23 points for every further melody-focused type of music stated as listened to. The number of harmony focused types of music appeared in the context of a positive dependency on the mean score progression in harmony training, increasing by 0.51 points for every further harmony-focused type of music stated as listened to. The time spent on passively listening to the type of music stated as most listened to increased mean harmony score by 0.13 points for every further hour spent on passively listening to the specified type of music per day. Both the number of harmony-focused types of music and the time spent on passively listening to the music most listened to failed to prove statistically significant explanatory variables.

See table 6-f below for a comprehensive overview of all explanatory variables for the tested score increase achieved during training with ToSCA. All tested potential variables which failed to prove as actually explanatory for one of the tested results were left out in the overview. The first value of the field indicates the gradient in the assumed linear context and the second one represents the p-value. The tested variables which proved to be explanatory are represented by the letters a through o in the overview with the following assignments: a) number of types of music stated as frequently listened to, b) participation in the type of music most listened to by singing a melody occurring in the music other than the main voice, c) participation in the music most listened to by singing a self-invented melody matching the music, d) no participation in the type of music most listened to by singing, e) number of different foci occurring with the types of music stated as frequently listened to, f) number of melody-focused types of music stated as frequently listened to, g) number of rhythm-focused types of music stated as frequently listened to, h) number of harmony focused types of music stated as frequently listened to, i) number of bi- or trifocal types of music stated as frequently listened to, j) musical focus of the type of music stated as most listened to being a bi- or trifocal type of music, k) participation in the music most listened to by drumming a rhythm occurring in the music other than the general beat, l) participation in the type of music most listened to by drumming a self-invented rhythm matching the music, m) no participation in the music most listened to by drumming or clapping along, n) hours spent on actively listening to the type of music stated as most listened to per day and o) hours spent on passively listening to the type of music stated as most listened to per day.

explanatory variable	mean pitch score increase	mean tempo score increase	mean melody score increase	mean rhythm score increase	mean harmony score increase	mean score increase
a)	0.37 0.007					0.76 0.13

b)	-038 0.34				1.50 0.006	
c)	0.51 0.29				2.11 0.007	
d)	0.69 0.12				1.20 0.03	
e)		0.31 0.07		-0.34 0.20		
f)			0.37 0.03		0.23 0.09	
h)				1.10 0.04	0.51 0.18	3.16 0.02
j)			-1.27 0.04			
k)			0.39 0.56	1.65 0.009		
l)			1.37 0.01	-0.17 0.69		
m)			0.86 0.19	0.02 0.97		
n)			-0.35 0.15			
o)					0.13 0.22	

table 6-f: influence of the subjects' musical habits on their mean score increase during aural training with ToSCA. First value: gradient in the assumed linear context. Second value: p-value.

The mean score increase for all categories proved most strongly dependent on the number of harmony-focused types of music, coinciding with a mean score progression raised by 3.16 points for every further harmony-focused type of music stated as listened to, revealing statistical significance with a p-value of 0.02. The total number of types of music stated as listened to appeared as another explanatory variable on the general score progression, which appears to increase by 0.76 points for every further type of music stated, however failing to prove statistically significant with a p-value of 0.13.

The number of harmony-focused types of music stated as listened to also proved a highly significant explanatory variable for the percentage of questions answered correctly in pitch training, which coincided with a rise of 6.48 points for every further harmony-focused type of music stated as listened to.

The percentage of questions answered correctly in tempo training proved dependent on the subjects' habits of drumming or clapping along to the music stated as most listened to. The drumming of a rhythm occurring in the music other than the general beat proved the strongest as well as a statistically significant explanatory variable, coinciding with a rise in the percentage of correct answers of 8.45 with a p-value of 0.04. The drumming of a self-invented rhythm matching the music appeared in the context of a positive dependency with the percentage of correct answers given in tempo training with an increase of 3.71 without any significant dependency. The lack of participation in the music stated as most listened to by drumming along proved another significant explanatory variable coinciding with a percentage of correct answers increased by 6.24 with a p-value of rounded-up 0.05.

The percentage of melody questions answered correctly in the course of training with ToSCA proved dependent on the participation in the music stated as most listened to by both singing along and drumming or clapping along. The lack of participation in the music by singing proved the strongest as well as a highly significant explanatory variable coinciding with the percentage of correctly answered melody questions increased by 15.67 at a p-value of 0.006. The singing along of a melody occurring in the music other than the main voice appeared in the context of a positive dependency with the percentage of correct answers raised by 0.69, whereas the singing of a self-invented voice matching the music appeared in the context of a negative dependency, with a decrease in the percentage of correct answers of 2.62, with both variables failing to prove statistically significant. The drumming along of a rhythm occurring in the music other than the general beat proved a positively correlated explanatory variable, coinciding with a rise in the percentage of correct answers in melody training of 12 and the drumming along of a self-invented rhythm matching the music coinciding with an increase in the correct answer percentage of 11.52. In contrast, the lack of participation in the music stated as most listened to by drumming or clapping along proved a negatively correlated explanatory variable, coinciding with a decrease in the percentage of correct answers given in melody training of 13.38, with the lack of participation in the music by drumming along and the drumming of a rhythm occurring in the music other than the general beat proving statistically significant explanatory variables and the drumming of a self-invented rhythm matching the music representing a highly significant explanatory variable with a p-value of 0.005.

The percentage of rhythm-questions answered correctly in the course of training with ToSCA also proved to be dependent on the participation in the music stated as most listened to by drumming or clapping along and by singing along. The drumming along of a rhythm occurring in the music other than the general beat proved the strongest and at the same time extremely highly significant explanatory variable for the percentage of correctly answered rhythm questions, coinciding with a rise of 19.19 at a p-value of 0.0005. The drumming along of a self-invented rhythm appeared in the context of a positive dependency, coinciding with an increase in the percentage of correct answers of 4.32, whereas the lack of participation in the music stated as most listened to by drumming was shown in the context of a negative dependency coinciding with a decrease in the percentage of correctly answered rhythm questions of 1.54, with neither of these two explanatory variables proving statistically significant. The participation in the music stated as most listened to by singing a melody occurring in the music other than the main voice revealed a strong trend towards a negative dependency on the percentage of correct answers coinciding with a decrease of 6.37 at a p-value of rounded-down 0.05. The singing along of a self-invented voice matching the music as well as the lack of participation in the music by singing along appeared as positively correlated explanatory variables, with the singing of a self-invented voice coinciding with a rise in the percentage of correct answers of 0.81 and the lack of participation in the music by singing coinciding with an increase in the correct answer percentage of 4.47. Both explanatory variables, however, failed to prove statistically significant.

The percentage of harmony questions answered correctly during training with ToSCA was shown to depend on the different music participation habits, the number of different types of music stated as listened to, the number of rhythm-focused types of music and the number of bi-or trifocal types of music stated as listened to. The drumming along of a rhythm occurring in the music other than the general beat proved the strongest and a highly significant explanatory variable, coinciding with a rise in the percentage of correctly answered harmony questions by 19.37 at a p-value of 0.003. The drumming along of a newly-invented rhythm matching the music proved another highly significant explanatory variable correlating with the percentage of correct answers raised by 11.54 at a p-value of 0.003. The lack of participation in the music by drumming or clapping, on the other hand, revealed a vague trend towards a negative correlation showing a decrease in the mean percentage of correct answers given in harmony training of 7.43. The lack of participation in the music by singing, however, proved a strong and significant explanatory variable coinciding with a rise in the percentage of correctly answered harmony questions by 13.52 at a p-value of 0.02. The participation in the music stated as most listened to by singing a melody occurring in the music other than the main voice and by singing a self-invented melody matching the music could be shown to be positively correlated explanatory variables as well with the singing of a self-invented voice coinciding with a rise in the mean percentage of correctly answered harmony questions by 11.72 and the singing of a voice occurring in the music other than the main voice coinciding with an increase in the mean percentage of correct answers by 5.14. Whereas the latter failed to prove a statistically significant explanatory variable, the singing of a self-invented voice was shown to be a statistically significant variable with a p-value of 0.01. The number of different types of music stated as listened to revealed a trend towards a negative correlation coinciding with a decrease in the mean percentage of correctly answered harmony questions by 4.12 for every further type of music stated as listened to. The number of bi- or trifocal types of music listened to proved a highly significant explanatory variable for the mean percentage of correct answers, which was shown to rise by 7.98 for every further bi- or tri-focal type of music stated as listened to at a p-value of 0.007. The number of rhythm-focused types of music appeared as a possible negatively correlated, but not significant, explanatory variable coinciding with a decrease in the mean percentage of correct answers given for harmony questions of 3.19.

The general percentage of questions answered correctly within all categories during training with ToSCA proved to be dependent on a large number of factors. Again, the participation in the music stated as most listened to by drumming along a rhythm occurring in the music other than the general beat proved the strongest and an extremely significant explanatory variable coinciding with an increase in the percentage of correct answers of 17.06 at a p-value of 0.0007. The p-values of 0.004 and 0.005 revealed a highly significant linear dependency on the participation in the music most listened to by drumming along of a self-invented rhythm, which coincided with a raise in the mean percentage of correct answers of 7.17, and the lack of participation in the music most listened to by drumming or clapping along, which concurred with a decrease in the mean percentage of correctly answered questions of 14. The lack of participation in the music most listened to by singing along proved a strong and highly significant explanatory variable, coinciding with a rise in the mean percentage of correct answers of 13.41 at a p-value of 0.002. The singing along of a melody occurring in the music other than the main voice revealed a trend towards being a negatively correlated explanatory variable for the mean percentage of correct answers, which appeared to decrease by 4.33. The singing along of a self-invented melody matching the music appeared as a possible negatively correlated linear regressor, concurring with a lowering of the mean percentage of correctly answered questions by 0.7, but remained without statistical significance. The number of different foci occurring with the types of music stated as listened to proved a negatively correlated and highly significant explanatory variable coinciding with a decrease in the mean percentage of correct answers of 6.02 at a p-value of 0.001. The number of different types of music stated as listened to appeared in the context of a decrease in the mean percentage of correct answers of 1.02, but failed to prove a statistically significant variable. Whereas the number of melody-focused types of music stated as listened to remained without any effect and the number of rhythm focused types of music listened to appeared as a possible, though statistically insignificant, explanatory variable concurring with a decrease in the mean percentage of correct answers of 0.89, the number of harmony-focused types of music listened to proved a strong and significant explanatory variable as well as the number of bi- or trifocal types of music revealing a strong and highly significant influence on the mean percentage of questions answered correctly during training with ToSCA. The number of harmony-focused types of music coincided with an increase in the percentage of correct answers of 6.54 for every further harmony-focused type of music stated as listened to at a p-value of 0.02 and the number of bi- or trifocal types of music listened to was shown to concur with a rise in the mean percentage of questions answered correctly of 6.06 for every further bi- or trifocal type of music stated as frequently listened to with a p-value of 0.003. The time spent on actively listening to the music stated as most listened to proved a positive and significant explanatory variable for the percentage of questions answered correctly in the course of training with ToSCA, whereas the time spent on passively listening to the music most listened to revealed a trend towards constituting a negatively correlated variable. The active music-listening time coincided with an increase in the mean percentage of correct answers of 3.23 for every further hour spent on actively listening to the type of music most listened to per day at a p-value of 0.01. The passive music-listening time, on the other hand, showed a trend towards being a negatively correlated variable, concurring with a decrease in the mean percentage of correctly answered questions of 0.78 for every further hour spent on passively listening to the type of music stated as most listened to per day.

See table 6-g below for a comprehensive overview of all factors influencing the tested percentages of questions answered correctly during training with ToSCA. Again, all tested potentially explanatory variables which failed to prove to be actually explanatory for one of the tested results were left out in the overview. The first value of the field indicates the degree of influence and the second value represents the p-value. The tested factors which proved to be influential are represented by the letters a through o in the overview with the above-specified assignments.[200]

200 cf. pages 92-93

explanatory variable	mean percentage of pitch questions answered correctly	mean percentage of tempo questions answered correctly	mean percentage of melody questions answered correctly	mean percentage of rhythm questions answered correctly	mean percentage of harmony questions answered correctly	mean percentage of total questions answered correctly
a)						-1.02 0.18
b)			-2.62 0.50	-6.37 0.05	5.14 0.14	-4.33 0.06
c)			0.69 0.88	0.81 0.82	11.72 0.01	-0.70 0.76
d)			15.67 0.006	4.47 0.27	13.52 0.02	13.41 0.002
e)					-4.12 0.07	-6.02 0.001
g)					-3.19 0.12	-0.89 0.35
h)	6.48 0.004					6.54 0.02
i)					7.98 0.007	6.06 0.003
k)		8.45 0.04	12.00 0.04	19.19 0.0005	19.37 0.003	17.06 0.0007
l)		3.71 0.17	11.52 0.005	4.32 0.14	11.54 0.003	7.17 0.004
m)		6.24 0.05	-13.38 0.02	-1.54 0.70	-7.43 0.10	-14.00 0.005
n)						3.23 0.01
o)						-0.78 0.08

table 6-g: influence of the subjects' musical habits on the mean percentage of questions answered correctly during aural training with ToSCA. First value: gradient in the assumed linear context. Second value: p-value.

The maximum score achieved during pitch training with ToSCA proved to be dependent on the number of types of music stated as listened to as well as on the subjects' participation in the music by singing along. The number of types of music listened to was shown to be a strong and highly significant explanatory variable for the maximum score achieved in pitch training, which was higher by 5.97 points for every further type of music stated as listened to. The subjects' habits of participating in the music most listened to appeared as further potential but not significant explanatory variables, with the singing along of a melody occurring in the music other than the main voice coinciding with a decrease in the maximum pitch score of 6.39 points, the singing along of a self-invented melody matching the music coinciding with an increase in the maximum pitch score of 8.34 points and the lack of participation in the music by singing coinciding with an increase in the maximum pitch score of 9.49 points.

The maximum score achieved during tempo training with ToSCA only revealed a trend towards a linear dependency on the number of harmony-focused types of music stated as listened to, which coincide with a rise in the maximum tempo score of 7.84 points for every further harmony-focused type of music stated as listened to.

The maximum score achieved in melody training was shown to be strongest and most significantly dependent on the subjects' participation in the music most listened to by drumming or clapping along of a self-invented rhythm matching the music, which concurred with an increase in the maximum melody score of 16.81 points at a p-value of 0.02. The drumming along of a rhythm occurring in the music other than the general beat and the lack of participation in the music most listened to by drumming or clapping along appeared as additional but non-significant explanatory variables, with the latter concurring with an increase in the maximum melody score of 7.6 points and the drumming along of a rhythm occurring in the music other than the general beat concurring with a raise in the maximum melody score of 5.61 points. Where the type of music stated as most listened to was a bi- or trifocal type of music, there was a vague trend towards a strong negative correlation coinciding with a decrease in the maximum melody score of 13.2 points.

The mean maximum score achieved in rhythm training with ToSCA proved to be dependent on both the subjects' participation in the music most listened to by singing and by drumming along as well as on the number of rhythm-focused and bi- or trifocal types of music listened to and the type of music most listened to being a bi- or trifocal type of music. Again, the drumming along of a rhythm occurring in the music other than the general beat proved the strongest and an extremely significant explanatory variable, coinciding with an increase in the maximum score achieved in rhythm training with ToSCA of 36.13 points at a p-value of 0.0005. The lack of participation in the music most listened to by drumming along revealed a trend towards a negative correlation, concurring with a decrease in the maximum rhythm score of 13.54 points and the drumming along of a self-invented rhythm matching the music appeared as a potential but non-significant explanatory variable, concurring with an increase in the maximum rhythm score of 5.49 points. The participation in the music most listened to by singing along rather than drumming along revealed a strong negative and significant correlation for the singing along of a melody occurring in the music other than the main voice, which coincided with a decrease in the maximum rhythm score of 11.9 points. The lack of participation in the music most listened to by singing along proved a strong and highly significant explanatory variable concurring with an increase in the maximum rhythm score of 19.63 points. The singing along of a self-invented melody matching the music appeared as an additional positive but non-significant explanatory variable, coinciding with an increase in the maximum rhythm score of 3.68 points. The number of rhythm-focused types of music proved a positive and significant explanatory variable, concurring with a rise in the maximum rhythm score of 4.16 points at a p-value of 0.04. Also the time spent on actively listening to the music stated as most listened to appeared as a positively correlated explanatory variable, coinciding with an increase in the maximum rhythm score of 3.15 points for every further hour spent on actively listening to the type of music most listened to, however failing to prove statistically significant.

The maximum score achieved in harmony training with ToSCA was shown to be dependent on a large number of factors, with the participation in the music most listened to by singing being the explanatory variable with the strongest effect. The singing along of a self-invented melody matching the music coincided with an increase in the maximum harmony score of 19.82 points, proving a highly significant linear regressor at a p-value of 0.005. The lack of participation in the music stated as most listened to by singing along proved a further strong and significant explanatory variable, concurring with a rise in the maximum harmony score of 18.76 points at a p-value of 0.02. The singing along of a melody occurring in the music other than the main voice revealed a trend towards coinciding with an increase in the maximum harmony score of 10.43 points. The p-values of 0.03 and 0.02, furthermore, revealed the participation in the music most listened to by drumming along of a rhythm occurring in the music other than the general beat, which coincided with an increase in the maximum harmony score of 16.5 points, and the drumming along of a self-invented rhythm matching the music, which concurred with an increase in the maximum harmony score of 10.79 points, as positive and significant explanatory variables for the maximum harmony score. The lack of participation in the music most listened to by drumming or clapping along, however, appeared as a potential but non-significant negatively correlated explanatory variable coinciding with a decrease in the maximum harmony score of 9.5 points. The type of music stated as most listened to being a bi- or trifocal type of music also appeared in the context of a negative correlation with the maximum score achieved in harmony training with ToSCA, coinciding with a decrease in the score of 7.41 points, though failing to prove statistically significant. The number of bi- or trifocal types of music listened to, however, proved a significant explanatory variable with a strong effect on the maximum harmony score, which was shown to rise by 8.55 points for every further bi- or trifocal type of music stated as listened to at a p-value of 0.01. The number of rhythm-focused types of music stated as listened to, on the other hand, appeared as a negatively correlated but non-significant linear regressor, concurring with a decrease in the maximum harmony score of 3.19 points for every further rhythm-focused type of music stated as listened to.

The summed up final score achieved in training with ToSCA was found to be dependent on the number of types of music stated as listened to and the number of rhythm-focused and harmony-focused types of music stated as frequently listened to. The number of harmony-focused types of music listened to proved a strong and significant explanatory variable coinciding with an increase in the final score of 48.17 points for every further harmony-focused type of music listened to. The total number of types of music listened to also revealed a strong and significant dependency, concurring with an increase in the final score of 20.34 points for every further type of music stated as frequently listened to. The number of rhythm-focused types of music listened to appeared as a potential negatively correlated but insignificant explanatory variable coinciding with a decrease in the final score of 17.62 points with every further rhythm focused type of music stated as frequently listened to.

See table 6-h below for a comprehensive overview of all explanatory variables for the tested maximum scores achieved during training with ToSCA. Once more, all tested potentially explanatory variables which failed to prove actually explanatory for one of the tested results were left out in the overview and again, the first value of the field indicates the degree of influence and the second value represents the p-value. The tested variables which proved to be explanatory are represented by the letters a through o in the overview with the above-specified assignments.[201]

explanatory variable	maximum pitch score	maximum tempo score	maximum melody score	maximum rhythm score	maximum harmony score	final total score
a)	5.97 0.003					20.34 0.02
b)	-6.39 0.28			-11.90 0.02	10.43 0.07	
c)	8.34 0.23			3.68 0.46	19.82 0.005	
d)	9.49 0.14			16.63 0.009	18.76 0.02	
f)			4.97 0.04			
g)				4.16 0.04	-3.19 0.28	-17.62 0.17
h)		7.84 0.08				48.17 0.01
i)					8.55 0.01	
j)			-13.20 0.10		-7.41 0.21	
k)			5.61 0.56	36.13 0.0005	16.50 0.03	
l)			16.81 0.02	5.49 0.16	10.79 0.02	
m)			7.60 0.36	-13.54 0.07	-9.50 0.16	
n)				3.15 0.20		

table 6-h: influence of the subjects' musical habits on the maximum scores achieved during aural training with ToSCA. First value: gradient in the assumed linear context. Second value: p-value.

6.3.4 Correlations between the Subjects' Self-Evaluation and Their Actual Test Performance

The subjects' impression of their own test performance was compared with their actual test results in terms of the percentages of final scores achieved in tests one and two, the percentages of questions answered correctly in tests one and two, the difference in score between test one and test two and the difference in the number of correct answers between test one and test two. The figures displaying the barplots of the subjects' answer frequencies in their self-evaluation and the graphs on the correlation between the subjects' self-evaluation and their actual test performance referred to in this subchapter are to be found in Appendices A.2 and A.3.

201 cf. pages 92-93

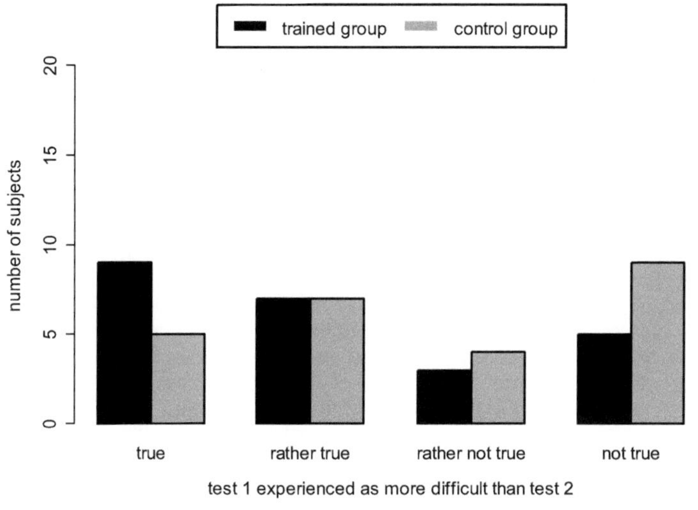

figure 6-17: answer frequencies for the statement of test 1 experienced as more difficult than test 2

As figure 6-17 shows, the first sound-discrimination test was experienced as more difficult than the second test by two thirds of the subjects participating in the aural training intervention between the two tests, as opposed to 48% of the control subjects experiencing the first test as more difficult. In figure A.3-66, the mean increase in the number of correct answers from test one to test two has been juxtaposed with the subjects' responses to the statement claiming that the first sound-discrimination test was more difficult than the second one. The decreasing graphs indicate a realistic self-evaluation by the subjects with the 9 subjects from the trained group confirming the statement as "true" being able to answer a mean of 3.89 more questions correctly than in the first test, as opposed to the 5 control-group subjects confirming the statement as "true", who were able to answer a mean of 2.6 more questions correctly in the second test. The subjects rejecting the statement as "not true" indeed suffered a decrease or a stagnation in the number of correct answers from the first to the second test, with a mean of -1.00 for the trained group and -0.11 for the control group. The mean increases in the number of correct answers given amounts to 1.29 for the trained-group subjects classifying the statement as "rather true" and to 2.86 for the control-group subjects responding to the statement with the same answer. The subjects categorising the statement as "rather not true" managed to achieve a small increase in the number of correct answers with a mean value of 0.67 for the trained group and 0.25 for the control group. As figure A.3-67 shows, the results in terms of the difference between the final scores achieved in test one and test two reveal less obvious correlations with the subject's estimation of their own performance. Whereas the two extreme responses of "true" and "not true" chosen by the trained-group subjects do represent both the largest score increase and the largest score decrease between the two tests, the middle responses of "rather true" and "rather not true" are interchanged in the subjects' self-evaluation. The mean score increases achieved by the trained group amount to 20.11 points for the subjects responding to the statement of the first sound-discrimination test being more difficult than the second by choosing the response option of "true", -0.14 points for the subjects responding with "rather true", 7.33 points for those choosing "rather not true" and -11.60 points for the subjects classifying the statement as "not true". The control group's responses correlate to the subjects' achieved score increase in terms of their categorising the statement as "true" and "rather true" in contrast to "rather not true" and "not true". However, in both cases, the mean score increases achieved by the subjects selecting one of the extreme response options and those achieved by the subjects responding with one of the middle options are interchanged. The subjects responding to the statement with "true" were able to increase their final test score by a mean of 8.40 points, those responding with "rather true" by a mean of 11.43 points, while those responding with "rather not true" suffered a decrease in their final test score by a mean of 6.00 points and those responding with "rather not true" were able to increase their final score by a mean of 4.67 points.

The second sound-discrimination test was experienced as more difficult than the first by two members of the trained group and four members of the control group as can be seen in figure A.2-46. Figures A.3-68 and A.3-69 display the correlation between the subjects' responses to the statement of the second test being more difficult than the first test and their achieved increase in the number of correct answers and the final score. As shown above, it was not possible to calculate mean values for the positive responses to the statement for the trained group since both the option of "true" and the option of "rather true" were selected by single subjects respectively with the subject responding with "true" in fact being able to answer 1 more question correctly and achieving a final score increased by 4 points in the second test. The subject responding with "rather true" in fact answered the same amounts of questions correctly in both tests while suffering a score decrease of 7 points in the second test as opposed to the final result achieved in the first test. The subjects who selected the response "rather not true" in fact suffered a mean decrease in the number of correct answers of 0.40 and a mean decrease in score of 3.40 points. The subjects rejecting the statement as "not true" were able to answer a mean of 0.64 more questions correctly and to achieve a final score increased by a mean of 9.65 points. For the control group, the only subject classifying the statement of the second sound-discrimination test being more difficult than the first one as "true" indeed suffered a decrease in the final score of 6.00 points, while still answering the same number of questions correctly in both tests. The control-group subjects responding with the opposite extreme of the statement being "not true", in fact, managed to achieve the lowest mean increase of 0.64 in the number of correct answers as opposed to a mean of 1.33 more correct answers given by the subjects classifying the statement as "rather true" and a mean of 2.86 more correct answers given by the subjects rejecting the statement as "rather not true". In terms of the increase in final scores, the control-group subjects selecting the statement response of "rather not true" were able to achieve a mean score increase of 3.33 points, indeed being lower than the mean score increase of the subjects selecting one of the negative response options. However, the mean score increase of the subjects responding with the extreme option of "not true" amounted to 4.50 points and was considerably lower than the mean score increase of 10.43 points achieved by the subjects who chose the milder response of "rather not true".

As can be seen in figures A.2-47, A.3-70 and A.3-71 indicating the response distribution for the statement of both sound-discrimination tests being equally difficult, where A.3-5 displays the correlation between the subjects' responses to this statement and their increase in the number of correct answers given in the second test as opposed to the first test and A.3-6 shows the correlation between the subjects' responses and their achieved score increases, the members of the trained group are more likely to classify both tests as equally difficult rather than the second test as more difficult in the case of lower achievement in the second test. The trained-group subjects who confirmed the statement as "true" in fact suffered a mean decrease in the number of correct answers of 1.67 and in the final score of 14.50 points. The control-group subjects who selected the extreme response of "true", on the other hand, indeed answered the same amount of questions correctly in both tests, but were however able to increase their final score by 7.14 points. The other responses of "rather true", "rather not true" and "not true" shall not be further investigated in this context because they apply for the two ambiguous contexts of either the first or the second test experienced as more difficult, which have already been discussed above.

With 58.33% of the trained group and 52% of the control group, the majority of subjects stated that they were not immediately able to adapt to the sound of the new language. As figure A.2-48 shows, only one subject per group confirmed the statement of immediately being able to adapt to the sound of the new language as "true", again making it impossible to average the actual percentage of the final score and the number of correct answers displayed in figures A.3-72 and A.3-73, in which the subjects' responses to the statement have been opposed to the mean percentage of final scores achieved and the mean percentage of questions answered correctly in test one. Figure A.3-72 indicates a coherent graph for the trained group with 77.40% of questions answered correctly for the subject having confirmed the statement as "true", a mean of 73.63% of questions answered correctly for the subjects confirming the statement as "rather true", a mean of 70.15% of questions answered correctly for the subjects rejecting the statement as "rather not true" and a mean of 69.99% of questions answered correctly for the subjects rejecting the statement as "not true". The percentages of the final score achieved by the trained group correlate fairly well with the subjects' impressions of their own performance as well, with only the mild and the extreme negative response being interchanged. In this context, the subject confirming the statement as "true" managed to achieve 68.70% of the possible score, the subjects confirming the statement as "rather true" achieved a mean of 64% of the possible score, the subjects rejecting the statement as "rather not true" achieved a mean of 60.97% of the maximum possible score and those rejecting the statement as "not true" achieved a mean of 62.11% of the possible score. For the control group, the true extreme values can be seen for the subjects who selected one of the middle responses rather than the extreme responses. The subject who confirmed the statement as "true" was able to answer 71.00% of the questions correctly and achieve 59.80% of the maximum possible score, the subjects confirming the statement as "rather true" managed to answer a mean of 76.29% of the questions correctly and to achieve a mean of 68.87% of the possible score, the subjects rejecting the statement as "rather not true" answered a mean of 69.04% of the questions correctly and achieved a mean of 58.96% of the maximum possible score and the subjects who rejected the statement as "not true" answered a mean of 72.36% of the questions correctly and achieved a mean of 64.01% of the maximum possible score.

As can be seen in figure A.2-49, 25% of the trained-group subjects and 48% of the control-group subjects confirmed the statement of being able to adapt to the sound of the new language in the course of the two tests as either "true" or "rather true". In figures A.3-74 and A.3-75, the subjects' responses to this statement have been opposed to the mean increases in the number of correct answers given from test one to test two and the mean increases in the scores achieved from test one to test two, expecting a decreasing graph with high mean increased values for subjects confirming the statement as true and decreased values of subjects who rejected the statement as not true. In fact, the graphs of both the trained and the control group reveal both the positive as well as the negative extreme within the two negative response options for both the increase in the number of correct answers and the increase in score. The subjects who rejected the statement as "not true" suffered a mean decrease in the number of correct answers of 1.40 and in the final score of 14.80 points in the case of the trained group and a mean decrease of 0.50 in the number of correct answers and 11.75 points in the final score in the case of the control group. The subjects who rejected the statement as "rather not true" on the other hand managed to answer a mean of 3.23 more questions correctly and to achieve a mean of 16.08 points more in the case of the trained group and to answer a mean of 2.67 more questions correctly and to achieve a mean of 15.89 points more in the case of the control group. Furthermore, the trained-group subjects who confirmed the statement as "true" were only able to answer a mean of 0.50 more questions correctly and suffered a mean decrease in the final score of 2.50 points, whereas the control-group subjects who confirmed the statement as "true" were able to answer a mean of 1.67 more questions correctly and to achieve a mean score increase of 4.00 points. The trained group subjects responding to the statement with "rather true" answered a mean of 3.23 more questions correctly and achieved a mean score increase of 3.50 points, similar to the control-group subjects who chose the "rather true" response achieving a mean score increase of 3.56 points and being able to answer a mean of 0.67 more questions correctly.

Figure A.2-50 shows that the majority of subjects did not feel that they were not able to adapt to the sound of the new language at all, with only 4 trained-group and 7 control-group subjects confirming the statement as "true" or "rather true". In figures A.3-76 and A.3-77, the subjects' responses to the statement have been juxtaposed with the percentage of questions answered correctly in the second test and the percentage of points achieved in the second test, expecting increasing graphs with low mean values for the subjects who chose positive responses and high values for the subjects who chose negative responses. For the responses of the trained group, the graphs reveal the positive extreme and the negative extreme in the two milder response options rather than in the extreme options, with the subjects confirming the statement as "rather true" answering a mean of 70.40% of the questions correctly and achieving a mean of 59.17% of the maximum possible score, as opposed to the subjects decisively confirming the statement as "true" answering a mean of 72.60% of the questions correctly and achieving a mean of 61.90% of the possible score. The subjects rejecting the statement as "rather not true" answered a mean of 76.68% of the questions correctly and achieved a mean of 69.97% of the maximum possible score as opposed to the subjects decisively rejecting the statement as "not true" answering a mean of 73.06% of the questions correctly and achieving a mean of 63.11% of the maximum possible score. The results of the control group reveal the smallest differences in the mean score and the mean number of correct answers for the two extreme response options, with the subjects confirming the statement as "true" answering a mean of 76.70% of the questions correctly and achieving a mean of 67.75% of the possible score and the subjects rejecting the statement as "not true" answering a mean of 76.24% of the questions correctly and achieving a mean of 67.58% of the possible score. Except for the high values achieved by the two subjects who chose the statement response of "true", the graphs indicate a realistic self-evaluation of the control-group subjects, with the subjects confirming the statement as "rather true" answering a mean of 70.96% of the questions correctly and achieving a mean of 60.02% of the possible score and the subjects rejecting the statement as "rather not true" answering a mean of 72.08% of the questions correctly and achieving a mean of 63.03% of the possible score.

As figure A.2-51 shows, the majority of subjects were able to remember sounds from the first test in the course of the second test with 79.17% of the members of the trained group and 92% of the members of the control group confirming the statement as either "true" or "rather true". In figures A.3-78 and A.3-79, the subjects' responses have been opposed to the mean increase values in the number of correct answers from test one to test two and the mean score increases in the second test as opposed to the first test expecting a decreasing graph with high values for the subjects confirming the statement and negative values for the subjects rejecting the statement. In fact, both extreme values are located within the negative responses in the graph representing the trained group for both the increase in the number of correct answers and the score increase. The subjects who rejected the statement as "rather not true" were able to answer a mean of 2.50 more questions correctly and to achieve a mean of 24.67 more points as opposed to the subjects decisively rejecting the statement as "not true", who suffered a decrease in the number of correct answers of 0.50 and a decrease in the final score of 13.50 points. The increases achieved by the trained-group subjects who confirmed the statement as true are located in between the values achieved by the subjects rejecting the statement, with the subjects who confirmed the statement as "rather true" answering a mean of 0.80 more questions correctly and achieving a mean of 5.80 more points and the subjects who decisively confirmed the statement as "true" answering a mean of 1.57 more questions correctly and achieving a mean score increase of 4.86 points. The control group's results indeed show a decreasing trend of the graph with a peak for the subjects who confirmed the statement and a decrease towards the subjects who rejected the statement, with the extreme negative response of "not true" not being selected at all within the control group. The mean increases for the subjects who responded with the milder positive option of "rather true" and for the subjects who responded with the extreme positive option of "true", however, are interchanged. The control-group subjects rejecting the statement as "rather not true" suffered a decrease in the number of correct answers by a mean of 2.50 and a mean score decrease of 16.50 points, as opposed to the subjects who confirmed the statement as "true" answering a mean of 0.77 more questions correctly and achieving a mean of 5.31 points more and the subjects confirming the statement as "rather true" answering a mean of 2.80 more questions correctly and achieving a mean score increase of 10.40 points.

For the inverse statement of the language sounds being completely different in the two tests, none of the subjects selected the extreme confirmative response option while the majority of subjects, with 87.5% of the members of the trained group and two thirds of the members of the control group rejected the statement as "not true", as shown in figure A.2-52. In this context, the subjects' responses were juxtaposed with their achieved mean increase in the number of correct answers from test one as opposed to test two and their mean score increase from the first to the second test expecting increasing graphs with negative values for the confirming response options and positive values for the rejecting response options. Figures A.3-80 and A.3-81, however, reveal opposing trends for the trained group and the control group, with the estimations of the control group showing the expected trend and the values of the trained group revealing a contrary trend. However, it has to be taken into account that the mean value for the trained-group subjects who confirmed the statement as "rather true" has been calculated from two subjects only and the value displayed for the rejecting response option of "rather not true" is a single value rather than a mean value, as opposed to the mean value formed by all other subjects of the trained group in the case of the extreme rejecting response of "not true". Except for one single control-group subject who selected the confirming response of "rather true", the distribution of answers is more representative for the control group, resulting in the expected graph direction. The control-group subjects decisively rejecting the statement as "not true" answered a mean of 1.56 more questions correctly and achieved a mean score increase of 7.63 points, as opposed to their results in the first test, while the trained-group subjects who selected the same response options answered a mean of 1.24 more questions correctly and increased their final score by a mean of 3.38 points.

Figure A.2-53 indicates that the majority of the subjects managed to recognise sound combinations from the first sound-discrimination test when taking the second test with two thirds of the trained group and 76% of the control group confirming this statement as either "true" or "rather true". In figures A.3-82 and A.3-83, the subjects' responses have been juxtaposed with their achieved increases in the number of correct answers given in test two as opposed to test one and the mean increase in the final scores achieved expecting decreasing graphs with high values for the subjects who confirmed the statement and negative values for the subjects rejecting the statement. In fact, the graph representing the increase in the number of correct answers for the trained group has its extremes at the middle response options with mean values contrary to those expected. The trained-group subjects who confirmed the statement as "rather true" only answered a mean of 0.25 more questions correctly and suffered a mean decrease in score by 0.25 points, whereas the subjects rejecting the statement as "rather not true" answered a mean of 4.25 more questions correctly and achieved a mean score increase of 19.00 points. The mean values indicated for the subjects who selected one of the extreme response options do not differ to a great extent, with the subjects confirming the statement as "true" answering a mean of 1.58 more questions correctly and achieving a mean of

5.17 more points and the subjects rejecting the statement as "not true" answering a mean of 1.00 more question correctly and achieving a mean score increase of 1.75 points. The expected graph direction could be seen with the graph indicating the control group's increase in the achieved scores, with the subjects decisively confirming the statement as "true" achieving a mean score increase of 12.36 points, the subjects confirming the statement as "rather true" achieving a mean of 3.25 more points and the subjects rejecting the statement as "rather not true" suffering a score decrease of 3.67 points. For the increase in the number of questions answered correctly by the control group, a similar but less obvious trend could be observed, with the subjects decisively confirming the statement as "true" answering a mean of 1.73 more questions correctly, the subjects confirming the statement as "rather true" giving a mean of 2.50 more correct answers and the subjects rejecting the statement as "rather not true" suffering a decrease in the number of correct answers of 1.00.

The inverse statement of the language-sound combinations of the second sound-discrimination test being completely different from the ones of the first test was rejected by all subjects except for one subject of the trained group and one subject of the control group who confirmed the statement as "rather true", as can be seen in figure A.2-54. Figures A.3-84 and A.3-85 juxtapose the subjects' responses with the respective groups' mean increases in the number of correct answers given in test two as opposed to test one and the mean score increase from the first to the second test expecting increasing graphs with high values for the subjects' decisively rejecting the statement as "not true". Leaving the single values displayed for the confirming response option of "rather true" unconsidered and focusing on the actually calculated mean values, the expected trend could be shown for both groups in terms of increase in the number of correct answers with a steeper increase for the control group. An even steeper increase can be observed for the control group's score increase, whereas the graph representing the trained group shows a mild decrease in this context. The trained-group subjects who rejected the statement as "rather not true" answered a mean of 0.33 more questions correctly and achieved a mean of 4.67 more points and the same group's subjects decisively rejecting the statement as "not true" answered a mean of 1.42 more questions correctly and achieved a mean score increase of 3.26 points. In contrast, the control-group subjects who rejected the statement as "rather not true" suffered a decrease in the number of correct answers of 5 and a mean score decrease of 27 points and the group's subjects who decisively rejected the statement as "not true" answered a mean of 2.05 more questions correctly and achieved a mean score increase of 9.10 points.

The first sound-discrimination test was experienced as extremely difficult with 45.83% of the members of the trained group and with 36% of the members of the control group confirming the statement as either "true" or "rather true", as shown in figure A.2-55. In figures A.3-86 and A.3-87, the subjects' responses to this statement have been juxtaposed with the percentage of questions answered correctly in test one and the score achieved in test one as a percentage of the highest possible score expecting increasing graphs with low mean values for subjects confirming the statement and high mean values for subjects rejecting the statement. As can be seen in figure A.2-55, the extreme response option of "true" was selected by only one single member of the control group and thus this value will be left unconsidered when regarding the correlation graphs. The expected positive trend from the confirming response options to the rejecting response options can be observed for both groups, with the results of the middle and the extreme positive response options being interchanged in the case of the trained group. The trained-group subjects who decisively confirmed the statement as "true" answered a mean of 63.97% of the questions correctly and achieved a mean of 52.07% of the possible score, the trained-group subjects who confirmed the statement as "rather true" answered a mean of 68.95% of the questions correctly and achieved a mean of 60.68% of the possible score, the subjects who rejected the statement as "rather not true" answered a mean of 76.14% of the questions correctly and managed to reach a mean of 68.12% of the maximum possible score and the subjects decisively rejecting the statement as "not true" gave a mean of 71.96% of correct answers and achieved a mean of 63.71% of the maximum possible score. The control-group subjects confirming the statement as "rather true" answered a mean of 68.95% of the questions correctly and achieved a mean of 76.20% of the maximum possible score, the control-group subjects who rejected the statement as "rather not true" answered a mean of 73.66% of the questions correctly and achieved a mean of 65.22% of the maximum possible score and the subjects selecting the response option of "not true" gave a mean of 75.05% of correct answers and achieved a mean of 66.10% of the maximum possible score.

The inverse statement of the first sound-discrimination test being extremely easy was rejected by all members of the trained group except for one and by 80% of the control group, as figure A.2-56 reveals. The graphs in figures A.3-88 and A.3-89 indicate the correlation between the subjects' selection of the four response options and the respective mean values for the percentage of questions answered correctly in test one and the mean percentage of the final scores achieved in test one in relation to the maximum score. The graphs were expected to show a negative trend with high values for subjects who selected the confirming response options and low values for subjects rejecting the statement. Again leaving the single values which could not be averaged unconsidered, the expected trend could be shown for both juxtapositions and for both groups, with the members of the trained group who rejected the statement as "rather not true" answering a mean of 75.46% of the questions correctly and achieving a mean of 67.28% of the maximum score and those members of the group decisively rejecting the statement as "not true" answering a mean of 69.18% of the questions correctly and achieving a mean of 60.38% of the possible score. The control-group subjects who confirmed the statement as "rather true" answered a mean of 74.60% of the questions correctly and achieved a mean of 66.90% of the maximum score, the control group's subjects who rejected the statement as "rather not true" answered a mean of 72.77% of the questions correctly and achieved a mean of 63.97% of the possible score and the subjects decisively rejecting the statement as "not true" answered a mean of 70.55% of the questions correctly and achieved a mean of 61.44% of the maximum score.

The statement of the second sound-discrimination test being experienced as extremely difficult was rejected by the majority of subjects with only 3 members of the trained group and 4 members of the control group classifying the statement as either "true" or "rather true", as displayed in figure A.2-57. In figures A.3-90 and A.3-91, the subjects' responses have been juxtaposed with the results achieved in the second sound-discrimination test expecting increasing graphs with low values for the subjects confirming the statement and high values for the subjects rejecting the statement. The expected trend, however, could only be observed for the general division of the subjects confirming the statement as opposed to the subjects rejecting the statement. In the case of the trained group, the mean value of the subjects who decisively rejected the statement as "not true" and the mean value of the subjects rejecting the statement as "rather not true" are interchanged as well as the mean values of the control-group subjects who strongly confirmed the statement as "true" and the control-groups subjects confirming the statement as "rather true". The mean percentages of questions answered correctly are 66.10% for the trained-group subjects and 69.45% for the control-group subjects who confirmed the statement as "true", 66.95% for the trained-group subjects and 66.10% for the control-group subjects confirming the statement as "rather true", 77.12% for the trained-group subjects and 74.36% of the control group subjects rejecting the statement as "rather not true" and 72.72% for the trained-group subjects and 77.85% for the control-group subjects rejecting the statement as "not true". The mean percentages of the maximum score achieved are 53.00% for the trained-group subjects and 57.25% for the control-group subjects who confirmed the statement as "true", 57.45% for the trained-group subjects and 56.55% for the control-group subjects who confirmed the statement as "rather true", 68.16% for the trained-group subjects and 65.35% for the control-group subjects rejecting the statement as "rather not true" and 63.46% for the trained-group subjects and 70.15% for the control-group subjects rejecting the statement as "not true".

The inverse statement of the second sound-discrimination test being extremely easy was confirmed as "true" by only 1 member per group and as "rather true" by 3 members per group, as displayed in figure A.2-58. In figures A.3-92 and A.3-93, the subjects' response choices were opposed to their results achieved in the second sound discrimination test in terms of the percentage of questions answered correctly and the percentage of the final score achieved expecting decreasing graphs with high mean values for the subjects confirming the statement and low mean values for those rejecting the statement. Once more leaving the single observations for the strongly confirmative response of "true" unconsidered, the expected trend could be shown for both the achieved score and the number of correct answers in both groups. The mean percentages of questions answered correctly are 80.10% for the trained-group subjects and 80.73% for the control-group subjects who confirmed the statement as "rather true", 73.81% for the trained-group subjects and 74.22% for the control-group subjects rejecting the statement as "rather not true" and 71.32% for the trained-group subjects and 71.44% for the control-group subjects strongly rejecting the statement as "not true". The mean percentages of the maximum score achieved are 74.47% for the trained-group subjects and 73.87% for the control-group subjects who confirmed the statement as "rather true", 63.54% for the trained-group subjects and 65.62% for the control-group subjects rejecting the statement as "rather not true" and 61.99% for the trained-group subjects and 60.69% for the control-group subjects strongly rejecting the statement as "not true".

The rather explicit statement of the achieved scores in both tests expected to be equal was confirmed by one third of the trained group as opposed to 52% of the control group as either "true" or "rather true", as shown in figure A.2-59. In figures A.3-94 and A.3-95, the subjects' responses have been opposed to the mean increase in score and in the number of correct answers given in the second sound-discrimination test as opposed to the first test. The main focus of this juxtaposition lies on the results of confirmative responses, which were expected to be close to 0. The results of the subjects rejecting the statement as "rather not true" or "not true" will remain unconsidered in this context due to the ambiguous statements behind the rejection of this specific statement. The statements of the score achieved in the first test expected to be higher and of the score achieved in the second test expected to be higher underlying the rejection of the above-issued statement will be examined separately in the following. As can be seen in figures A.3-94 and A.3-95, however, the trained-group subjects who confirmed the statement as "true" suffered a mean decrease in the number of correct answers given in test two as opposed to test one by 4.50 and an extreme mean score decrease of 39 points as opposed to the control-group subjects who confirmed the statement as "true", who were able to answer a mean of 2.6 more questions correctly and to achieve a mean of 13.8 more points in the second test as opposed to the first test. The trained-group subjects who confirmed the statement less decisively as "rather true" answered a mean of 0.83 more questions correctly and achieved a mean of 1.33 more points, as opposed to the control-group subjects who confirmed the statement as "rather true", who were able to answer a mean of 0.80 more questions correctly and to achieve a mean of 5.50 more points.

The statement of a better score expected for the first sound-discrimination test as opposed to the second one was confirmed as "true" by 1 subject of the trained group and 2 subjects of the control group and as "rather true" by 1 subject of the trained group and 3 subjects of the control group only, as figure A.2-60 indicates. Figures A.3-96 and A.3-97 juxtapose the mean increase in the number of correct answers and the mean score increase with the subjects' responses to this statement. In this context, increasing graphs with negative values for the subjects confirming the statement and positive values for the subjects rejecting the statement were expected. When leaving out the single observations occurring for the response options of "true" and "rather true" within the trained group, the expected increasing graph could be seen. However, the mean of results achieved by the subjects rejecting the statement as "rather not true", contrary to the expectations, lies below the zero mark. The expected graph direction could be observed for the control group with an exception of the results achieved by the two subjects confirming the statement as "true", who were, in fact, able to achieve a score rise of 16.50 points and an increase in the number of correct answers of 3.50. The trained group subjects rejecting the statement as "rather not true" answered a mean of 0.20 fewer questions correctly and suffered a mean score decrease of 2.40 points as opposed to the trained-group subjects more decisively rejecting the statement as "not true", who were able to answer a mean of 2.24 more questions correctly and to achieve a mean of 7.65 more points in the second test as opposed to the first test. The control-group subjects who confirmed the statement as "rather true" indeed suffered a mean decrease in the number of correct answers of 2.00 and in the achieved score of 8.33 points, whereas the control-group subjects rejecting the statement as "rather not true" were able to raise their score by a mean of 2.00 points and their number of correct answers by a mean of 1.25. The subjects rejecting the statement as "not true" managed to increase their number of correct answers by a mean of 1.83 and their achieved score by a mean of 9.67 points.

The inverse statement of a higher score expected for the second sound-discrimination test as opposed to the first test was confirmed by 56.52% of the trained group and 50% of the control group, as shown in figure A.2-61. In figures A.3-98 and A.3-99, the subjects' responses were opposed to the mean increase in the number of correct answers and the mean score increase achieved from the first to the second sound-discrimination test expecting decreasing graphs with positive values for the subjects confirming the statement and negative values for the subjects rejecting the statement. Leaving out the single observation of only one control-group subject who responded to the statement with "true", the graphs show the expected trend for the middle response options of "rather true" and "rather not true" while experiencing a steep and unexpected increase between the two negative response options. The subjects who confirmed the statement as "true" answered a mean of 3.00 more questions correctly in the second test in the case of the trained group and did not show any improvement in the number of correct answers in the case of the control group, the subjects confirming the statement as "rather true" answered a mean of 0.40 questions more correctly in the case of the trained group and a mean of 3.40 more questions in the case of the control group, the subjects who rejected the statement as "rather not true" answered a mean of 0.40 fewer questions correctly in the case of the trained group and a mean of 2.67 fewer questions in the case of the control group and those subjects rejecting the statement as "not true" answered a mean of 2.75 more questions correctly in the case of the trained group and a mean of 2.14 more questions in the case of the control group. The score increase achieved by the subjects who confirmed the statement as "true" amounts to 13.60 points for the trained group and 1.50 points for the control group, the score increase achieved by the subjects confirming the statement as "rather true" averages out at 1.20 points for the trained group and 13.10 points for the control group, the subjects rejecting the statement as "rather not true" suffered a mean score decrease of 10.00 points in the case of the trained group and of 14.33 points in the case of the control group. Finally, the subjects decisively rejecting the statement as "not true" were able to increase their final score by a mean of 13.00 points in the case of the trained group and by 13.14 points in the case of the control group.

The statement of a good score being expected for the first sound-discrimination test was confirmed as either "true" or "rather true" by 30.43% of the trained group and one third of the control group, as shown in figure A.2-62. In figures A.3-100 and A.3-101, the subjects' responses have been juxtaposed with their achievement in the first sound-discrimination test in terms of the percentage of questions answered correctly and the percentage of the maximum score achieved expecting decreasing graphs with high values for the subjects confirming the statement and lower values for the subjects rejecting the statement. Once again leaving out the single observation of only one member of the trained group who selected the "true" response option, the graphs for the trained group show almost identical mean values for the subjects selecting the middle response options and a lower value for those rejecting the statement as "not true". The graphs indicating the control group's results have both their positive and their negative extremes within the positive response options revealing an unexpected increasing direction for the negative response options. The percentage of questions answered correctly by subjects who confirmed the statement as "true" amounts to 76.33% for the control group, the percentages of questions answered correctly by subjects confirming the statement as "rather true" amount to 71.50% for the trained group and 68.08% for the control group, the subjects rejecting the statement as "rather not true" answered a mean of 71.75% of the questions correctly in the case of the trained group and a mean of 72.18% in the case of the control group and the subjects strongly rejecting the statement as "not true" answered a mean of 70.39% questions correctly in the case of the trained group and a mean of 72.60% in the case of the control group. At the same time, the mean score achieved by the control-group subjects who selected the response option of "true" amount to 69.30% of the maximum score, the mean score of subjects confirming the statement as "rather true" amounts to 62.98% of the possible score for the trained group and 58.70% for the control group, the score achieved by subjects who selected the "rather not true" response option averages out at 63.31% of the maximum score for the trained group and 63.50% for the control group and the mean score achieved by the subjects who strongly rejected the statement as "not true" amounts to 61.53% of the maximum possible score for the trained group and 63.23% for the control group.

The statement of a high score being expected for the second sound-discrimination test was confirmed by 56.52% of the trained group and 50% of the control group, as displayed in figure A.2-63. Figures A.3-102 and A.3-103 juxtapose the subjects' responses to the statement with their test results achieved in the second sound-discrimination test expecting decreasing graphs with high values for the subjects confirming the statement and lower values for the subjects rejecting the statement. The expected trend could be shown for the control group with interchanged results within the negative response options. The trained group revealed the expected graph direction with an exception of unexpectedly low mean values for the subjects who decisively confirmed the statement as "true" amounting to a mean percentage of correctly answered questions of 71.94% and a mean percentage of the maximum score of 62.90% as opposed to the control group's result in the same response category averaging out at 82.30% of the questions answered correctly and 74.70% of the possible score achieved. The subjects who confirmed the statement less decisively as "rather true" achieved a mean percentage of correct answers of 78.06% for the trained group and 75.26% for the control group and a mean percentage of the maximum score of 69.91% for the trained group and 47% for the control group. The mean percentages of questions answered correctly by subjects rejecting the statement as "rather not true" amount to 72.64% for the trained group and 71.61% for the control group and the mean percentage of the maximum score to 63.62% for the trained group and 61.64% for the control group. The subjects who decisively rejected the statement as "not true" achieved a mean percentage of correct answers of 69.66% in the case of the trained group and 73.38% in the case of the control group and a mean percentage of the maximum possible score of 58.50% in the case of the trained group and 64.13% in the case of the control group.

The statement of a low score being expected for the first sound-discrimination test was confirmed by a fourth of the members of the trained group and a fifth of the members of the control group as either "true" or "rather true", as shown in figure A.2-64, with the response option of "true" not being selected by any of the control-group subjects. In figures A.3-104 and A.3-105, the subjects' responses to this statement were opposed to their actual test results in the second sound-discrimination test in terms of the percentage of questions answered correctly and the percentage of the maximum possible score achieved, expecting increasing graphs with low mean values for subjects confirming the statement and higher mean values for subjects rejecting the statement. The expected trend could be shown for the graphs indicating the trained group's results as opposed to the graphs indicating the control group's results, which have their positive as well as their negative extreme with the middle response options in decreasing direction rather than the expected increase. The trained-group subjects managed to answer a mean of 67.75% of the questions correctly when confirming the statement as "true", a mean of 68.53% of the questions when confirming the statement as "rather true", a mean of 70.68% of the questions when rejecting the statement as "rather not true" and a mean of 72.18% of the questions when decisively rejecting the statement as "not true". The percentages of questions answered correctly by the control group average out at 72.92% for subjects confirming the statement as "rather true", 71.78% for subjects rejecting the statement as "rather not true" and 71.89% for subjects strongly rejecting the statement as "not true". The percentages of the maximum score achieved by the trained group add up to means of 59.45% for subjects confirming the statement as "true", 59.70% for subjects confirming the statement as "rather true", 61.68% for subjects rejecting the statement as "rather not true" and 63.68% for subjects rejecting the statement as "not true". The control group achieved mean score percentages of 64.26% for subjects confirming the statement as "rather true", 61.83% for subjects rejecting the statement as "rather not true" and 63.19% for subjects strongly rejecting the statement as "not true".

The statement of a low score being expected for the second sound-discrimination test was rejected by 75% of the trained-group subjects and by 68% of the control-group subjects, as shown in figure A.2-65, with none of the subjects of either group having selected the extreme confirmative response option of "true". In figures A.3-106 and A.3-107, the subjects' responses to the statement were juxtaposed with their actual test results in the second sound-discrimination test expecting increasing graphs with low mean values for the subjects confirming the statement and higher mean values for the subjects rejecting the statement. The expected trends could be observed for the trained group in correlation with the subjects' achieved scores and less obviously for the correlation with the subjects' percentage of correctly answered questions, which experiences a slight decrease between the two negative response options. With the control group, the expected trend is interrupted by the unexpectedly low mean value of the subjects who selected the "rather not true" response option. The trained-group subjects who confirmed the statement as "rather true" answered a mean of 70.15% of the questions correctly and achieved a mean percentage of the maximum possible score of 58.70% as opposed to the control-group subjects responding to the statement in the same way, who answered a mean of 73.17% of the questions correctly and achieved a mean percentage of the maximum score of 64.03%. The trained-group subjects who rejected the statement as "rather not true" answered a mean of 74.25% of the questions correctly and achieved a mean percentage of the maximum score of 64.15%, whereas the control-group subjects who responded to the statement in the same way answered a mean of 68.08% of the questions correctly and achieved a mean percentage of the maximum score of 57.50%. Whereas the trained-group subjects strongly rejecting the statement as "not true" answered a mean of 73.86% of the questions correctly and achieved a mean percentage of the maximum score of 64.93%, the control-group subjects who selected this response option answered a mean of 76.22% of the questions correctly and achieved a mean percentage of the maximum score of 67.62%.

6.4 Discussion

The main hypothesis of the present study expecting increased test results in the second sound-discrimination test as opposed to the first test proved true to the extent that the achieved final scores improved significantly for the mean of all subjects as well as, separately, for the trained group, whereas the expected effect on the number of correct answers given by all subjects remained insignificant. Furthermore, the comparison between the mean score increase and the mean increase in the number of correct answers given by the trained group and by the control group failed to reveal significant differences. Even though the trends towards a potential influence of ToSCA on the results achieved in the post-intervention sound-discrimination test are obvious, the expected effect could not be shown with significant differences from the results achieved by the control group. This leads to the supposition that the time of interventive treatment applied in the present context does not suffice in order to cause any considerably significant differences. In sum, fourteen training sessions of fifteen minutes per day only amount to three and a half hours of interventive measures in a period of two weeks. Further studies will have to show whether the trend revealed here can be corroborated by more significant results after a longer training period. The potential of the program, comprising tens of thousands of possible questions, was nowhere near exhausted by any of the subjects during the training time, so the program is well suited for much longer training periods, which unfortunately were not practicable in the course of the present study due to the subjects' voluntary and unpaid participation, the workload for which had to remain within reasonable limits to allow for a sufficient number of participants.

The comparison between the result differences achieved by the trained group and by the control group did not reveal any significant differences between the two groups. The two categories of difficulty-grade-four questions which revealed a trend towards a better increase in favour of the trained group and difficulty-grade-six questions which showed a tendency towards a better increase in favour of the control group appear extremely random in the context of the obtained results. The expected distinctly beneficial effect on the performance of the trained group in the questions of higher difficulty could not be shown.

In close examination of the influence of the single ToSCA training fields on the single test categories queried in the course of the sound-discrimination tests, the most significant results were obtained for an apparently negative correlation between the percentage of pitch questions answered correctly and the ability to locate a word in a sentence. The test categories on the location of a word in a sentence as well as the number of words in a sentence, the word heard at a certain slot of the sentence and the word order in a sentence were hypothesised to be positively influenced by training in the duration of sounds, i.e. rhythm and tempo, rather than by the space-oriented training categories of pitch, melody and harmony. Negative correlations as shown at a high level of significance for the above-described pairing, even though unexpected, are not contradictory to the assumed affinities in the context of tone duration in contrast to tone space. The same test category on the location of a word in a sentence proved significantly dependent on a set of other training fields of ToSCA. Whereas a negative correlation was shown between the percentage of pitch questions answered correctly and the ability to locate a word in a sentence, this specific test-question category appeared to be positively dependent on the maximum score achieved in the very same ToSCA training category of pitch. This leads to the conclusion that a large number of pitch questions answered, whether correctly or incorrectly, is more beneficial for the ability to locate a word in a sentence than the careful consideration of answer choices in order to make sure to select the correct answer option. The expected positive correlation between the ability to locate a word in a sentence and the subjects' achievements in tempo training with ToSCA in fact proved a minor but significant negative correlation with the number of correct answers given in this test category. The percentage of rhythm questions answered correctly, however, did show the expected positive effect at a high level of significance. The fact that this test-question category furthermore proved significantly positively dependent on the maximum score achieved during harmony training leads to the conclusion that the original differentiation between tempo and rhythm as time-oriented aural training fields and pitch, melody and harmony as space-oriented aural training areas is too rough for a precise description of the beneficial effects of the different musical training categories on the different tested aspects of sound discrimination. Most test-question categories proved to be dependent on more than one factor, often intermingling time- and space-oriented training areas, which underlines the importance of a complete training in all potential factors.

Other than the above-described influential relationships, only two more significant effects could be shown as influences on the maximum score achieved during tempo training. A positive effect of a high score and a high number of correct answers in the training field of tempo on the ability to identify the number of words in a sentence was expected and the hypothesis could be confirmed by the results. The negative effect of the same training category on the ability to identify a heard word in writing is not contradictory to the expectation in so far as this test-question category was expected to depend on the subjects' performance in the space-oriented fields of training. However, a positive effect of the space-oriented training areas was expected rather than a negative correlation between the ability to identify a heard word in writing and the time-oriented training areas. At the same time, the subjects' performance in pitch training, as one of the space-oriented training areas, reveals a positive correlation with this training field.

Furthermore, two opposing trends could be seen for the question category testing the ability to identify the word heard at a certain slot of the sentence, which was expected to be dependent on the space-oriented training fields of aural training. Here, the study revealed a positive correlation with the percentage of rhythm questions answered correctly during training with ToSCA but also a positive correlation with the maximum score achieved in melody training, with the effect of melody training showing a stronger impact than the effect of rhythm training.

As expected, the test-question category dealing with the identification of a heard sentence in writing revealed a trend towards a positive correlation with the percentage of melody questions answered correctly. Additionally, a negative but insignificant correlation with the maximum score achieved in tempo training could be observed.

To sum up the correlations between the results achieved in the single training categories of ToSCA and the performance enhancement achieved in the single test-question categories of the second sound-discrimination test as opposed to the first one, the predictions made for the identification of the number of a words in a sentence depending on the performance in the time-oriented training fields of ToSCA and for the identification of written input in acoustic form depending on the performance in the space-oriented training fields of the aural training program proved true, whereas the predicted dependencies for the identification of word locations in sentences proved more complex than expected and no significant dependencies could be found for the test-questions dealing with the identification of a heard word in writing, the identification of the word order in a sentence and the identification of the word differing in the written representation of a sentence from its acoustic representation. It may be concluded that tasks dealing with the location of words in sentences, comprising the two test-question types dealing with the identification of a word heard at a certain slot of a sentence and the location of a word in a sentence, are dependent on both time- and space-oriented abilities with the time-oriented abilities taking care of the actual localisation task and the space-oriented abilities in charge of mental preconceptions of the sound of the word sought after. The tasks testing the ability to identify the number of words in a sentence, on the other hand, do not require any such sound-preconception abilities and seem to exclusively rely on the time-oriented aspects of listening skills. The task types which test the ability to identify a written word or sentence in acoustic form appear to be the other extreme, depending on mental sound-preconception abilities while not requiring any time-oriented sound-discrimination skills.

The dependence of the subjects' test performances on their previous language-learning and application experience revealed some interesting correlations. In contrast to the initially expected correlations, no dependency could be shown for the results achieved in the first sound-discrimination test, apparently leaving all previous language experience insignificant in the context of the initial test performance. However, the performance enhancement from the first to the second sound-discrimination test proved strongly dependent on the number of foreign languages used in every-day life, which was an expected dependency. Other factors such as the number of languages learned at school and the number of languages learned in a voluntary out-of school context were not found to be influential.

The hypothesised differences in results during training with ToSCA proved true in terms of subjects with an affinity for rhythm-focused types of music achieving a notably higher total score in the rhythm-training category than other subjects and subjects with an affinity for melody-focused types of music achieving a considerably higher maximum score in the melody-training category than other subjects. Additionally, the mean melody-score increase between the single sessions was significantly higher for subjects with a preference for melody-focused music than for subjects with other musical preferences. The further hypothesised effects of an affinity towards melody-focused types of music on the results in pitch training and of an affinity towards rhythm-focused types of music on the results in tempo training could not be shown. As expected, subjects with a preference for multi-focal types of music achieved significantly higher maximum scores and a considerably higher percentage of correct answers in the training category of harmony as well as in the entire number of correct answers. This confirms the assumption that subjects' usual music-listening preferences would influence their receptivity to and performance in the different training fields of ToSCA. In a further study, it may be interesting to compare the results of subjects with a preference for types of music with the same musical focus.

The subjects' participation in the music listened to by drumming or singing along was hypothesised to be more beneficial for the final results achieved in ToSCA the more creative or musically advanced the level of participation is, with no participation being least beneficial and the singing of the main voice or the drumming of the general beat, the singing of a different voice from the music or the drumming of a rhythm occurring in the music and the invention of a new voice or rhythm matching the music being more beneficial respectively. These hypotheses, however, could not be confirmed as such. The only significant result for the influence of participation in the music by singing was oddly found for the subjects who stated that they did not take part in the music by singing, the option of which proved the most beneficial in the context of the percentage of correct answers in melody training. The expected results for the subjects' participation by singing were surprisingly found in the harmony-training category instead, with the best mean score increase from one training session to the next and the best maximum score achieved by subjects having stated to sing a newly invented voice matching the music. This may seem self-explanatory in retrospect, since the invention of a new melody matching the music naturally requires a mental conception of and feeling for the harmonic procedure of the piece of music in question. The hypotheses on the participation in the music listened to by drumming along only proved true in terms of a participation in the music by drumming or clapping along being more beneficial than a lack of participation. The strongest results were obtained for the subjects who stated that they drum a rhythm occurring in the music other than the general beat as opposed to an apparent negative effect of the lack of participation on the subjects' achievement in rhythm training. The expected high results for those subjects who stated that they invent a new rhythm matching the music could not be shown.

The expected positive effect of a high number of hours per day spent on actively listening to music on the subjects' performance in the training with ToSCA could be shown for the percentage of correct answers, which proved significantly higher for every further hour of active music listening, but not for the maximum scores achieved in the course of the training. This may lead to the conclusion that subjects with the habit of extensive and attentive listening are more likely to take enough time to answer questions correctly and thus, in total, work on fewer questions than other subjects.

In contrast to the above-discussed results, the expected beneficial effect of a high number of different types of music stated as listened to on the maximum score and the percentage of questions answered correctly proved contrary. For every further type of music stated as listened to, the percentage of questions answered correctly proved significantly lower. This does not reveal the expected effect of a high number of different types of music listened to indicating a high receptivity towards the music used within ToSCA. On re-examination of the original survey data, this turn towards an unexpected result can be explained by the subjects having stated to listen to a large number of different kinds of music revealing a tendency towards stating very specific subgenres of one general genre such as rock music, whereas those subjects with a wider interest tend to indicate the main genres such as jazz, rock or classical music rather than stating inter-genre nuances with very specific designations. So the plain number of types of music stated as listened to does not contribute to the analysis of beneficial factors in the present context. This might raise the expectations for the results on the influence of the amount of different musical foci occurring in the types of music stated as listened to, which unfortunately failed to prove an influential factor after all.

The expected beneficial effect of a high number of languages learned in a school context and a high number of languages learned in a voluntary out-of-school context could neither be shown for the final results of the first sound-discrimination test in terms of the final score or the number of correct answers nor for the score improvement or the progression of correct answers in the second as opposed to the first test. Thus the furthermore expected better beneficial effect of a high number of languages learned in a voluntary context as opposed to a high number of languages learned in an obligatory context on the perceptive performance in the tested language could not be shown either. On a more specific level, a high number of languages learned in a voluntary context even proved counterproductive for the score progression as well as for the progression in the number of correct answers for the identification of a word heard at a certain slot of a sentence and the identification of the word in a sentence deviating in the written form of the sentence from its acoustic representation. A negative progression from the first to the second test in these two specific categories may be explained by the fact that neither of the learned languages bears any resemblance to the tested language. Furthermore, the clear majority of languages stated as learned belongs to the Romanic and the Germanic linguistic families, so a high number of learned languages with identical origin seems to manifest a certain preconception of how a foreign language is structured. Why this effects these two aspects of language perception, while leaving others, which may differ to a greater extent from Romanic and Germanic language, unaffected cannot be satisfactorily answered by means of the present data. The positive progression for the performance in questions on the identification of a heard word in writing in the second sound-discrimination test as opposed to the first one, surprisingly proved stronger for those subjects who had learned many languages in an obligatory context than for those subjects who had learned many languages in a voluntary context but nevertheless is distinct for both. In total, the better beneficial effect of a high number of languages learned in a voluntary context as opposed to a high number of languages learned in an obligatory context could not be shown.

The above-described negative performance progression from the first to the second sound-discrimination test in the identification of the word in a sentence differing in the written form of the sentence from its acoustic representation can also be found in the context of years spent on language learning. This again underlines the theory of a fixed preconception of a language's structure within the subjects who had learned several languages from the same linguistic family. Furthermore, the performance in questions on the identification of a heard word in written form also showed a positive progression from the first to the second sound-discrimination test.

The years elapsed since the subjects' last language-learning activity failed to show the expected effect on the total test results in the first test and the performance progression from the first to the second test. In the specific case of the above-discussed questions on the identification of the word differing in the written form of a sentence from its acoustic representation, it could be shown that the more time elapsed since the subject's last language-learning activity, the worse the performance progression from the first to the second test became in this test category. This may seem contradictory regarding the above-described results on first glance. However, if the structure and composition of a language are the aspects most remembered, these data again underline the theory of the structural language preconception developed by the learner of languages with identical linguistic origin.

The number of languages currently used by the subjects was the only factor distinctly revealing a positive effect on the total performance progression from the first to the second sound-discrimination test. As originally hypothesised, the more languages currently used by the subject, the higher the subjects' receptivity towards a new language and thus a strong progression could be shown especially in terms of score improvement in the second sound-discrimination test as opposed to the first one for subjects currently using a high number of foreign languages in every-day life. Beneficial effects could especially be shown for questions on the identification of a word heard at a specific slot of a sentence, the word order of a sentence and the identification of a written sentence in acoustic form. All of these task types focus on the sentence level of language, which may lead to the conclusion that subjects using a high number of foreign languages daily seem to be more able to deal with longer passages of unknown words without losing track of the heard or read parts of speech.

The expected trend in the context of self-evaluation of the trained group being more likely to select the extreme answer options of "true" or "not true" than the control group proved true for all statements except for two. 58% of the trained group's subjects decided for one of the extreme answer options when responding to the statement "I think I answered hardly any question correctly in the first sound-discrimination test." as opposed to 64% of the control group's subjects. The statement "The sound combinations from the first and second sound-discrimination tests were completely different." was met with one of the extreme responses by 82.6% of the trained group's subjects, as opposed to 87.5% of the control group's subjects. It may be concluded that statements on details of the first sound-discrimination test are more difficult to evaluate for subjects who have been taking part in extra interventional activities between the two tests, so the expected trend towards more decisive answer options could not be shown for these special statements.

The hypothesis on the trained group's subjects classifying their performance in the second sound-discrimination test as better than in the first test could be verified, with 62.5% of the trained group's subjects stating their impression of having answered more questions correctly in the second test than in the first test, as opposed to 48% of the control group's subjects. The statement "I think I answered the same number of questions correctly in both sound-discrimination tests." was confirmed as "true" or "rather true" by 52% of the control group, as opposed to one third of the trained group, as expected. Correspondingly, the first sound-discrimination test was experienced as more difficult than the second one by a slight majority of again 52% of the control group's subjects and a clear majority of two thirds of the trained group's subjects, again as expected. The hypothesis on the evaluation of the grade of difficulty proved true as well, with 45.8% of the trained group's subjects classifying the first sound-discrimination test as extremely difficult, as opposed to only 12.5% classifying the second test as extremely difficult. The first test was also experienced as extremely difficult by 36% of the control group's subjects, while only 16.6% stated the same for the second test.

The hypothesised correspondence of the subjects' stating their immediate accustomisation to the sound of the new language with a good performance in the first sound-discrimination test already only proved true for the trained group. The control group's subjects who classifyed the statement as "rather true" revealed a better understanding of the language than those decisively classifying the statement as "true".[202] The expected correlation between the subjects' evaluation of their test performance as having gradually gotten used to the sound of the new language and their improvement in score and the number of correct answers from the first to the second test could not be shown. Even though the mean of subjects classifying the statement as "true" did show an improvement and the mean of subjects rejecting the statement as "not true" showed a decrease in the number of correct answers for both groups, the mean of subjects rejecting the statement as "rather not true" achieved the best improvement in the number of correct answers for both the trained and the control group.[203] Also the graphs on the correlation between the subjects' evaluation of their gradual accustomisation to the sound of the new language and their score increase from the first to the second sound-discrimination test revealed peaks for the groups of subjects rejecting the statement as "rather not true" for the trained group as well as the control group.[204] In this context, it may be argued that the gradual accustomisation to the sound of a language is a term which does not specify any specific point of time, so a slow gradual accustomisation to the sounds of the language will certainly achieve different results than a quick accustomisation. The subjects' response to the statement of not having been able to get accustomed to the sound of the new language only partially met the expected correlation towards the achieved score and number of correct answers in the second sound-discrimination test. Contrary to the hypothesis, the control group's subjects who decisively confirmed the statement as "true" achieved a better mean in the final score as well as in the number of correct answers than any of the other answer options' mean values, which, however, show a rising graph from "rather true" up to "not true" as expected. The trained group's subjects were most realistic in their evaluation when responding to the statement with one of the middle options of "rather true" or "rather not true" for both the final score and the number of correct answers given in the second sound-discrimination test.[205]

The subjects' response to the statements directly comparing the two sound-discrimination tests could only partially show the expected correlation with their actual performance and performance progression. Whereas the statement of the first test being experienced as more difficult than the second test did show declining graphs for both groups in the score progression as well as the increase in the number of correct answers[206], the correlation graphs on the reverse statement of the second sound-discrimination test being experienced as more difficult than the first

202 cf. figure A.3-72 in Appendix A.3
203 cf. figure A.3-74 ibid.
204 cf. figure A.3-75 ibid.
205 cf. figures A.3-76 and A.3-77 in Appendix A.3
206 cf. figures A.3-66 and A.3-67 ibid.

one appeared contradictory for the two groups.[207] Neglecting the graph points representing the two answer options of "true" and "rather true" for the trained group, which represent absolute values rather than mean values due to the options having been selected by only one subject respectively, the subjects' self-evaluation appears realistic in the sense of the mean of subjects who decisively rejected the statement as "not true" representing the peak of the graph. The graph point indicating the mean of the trained group's subjects who rejected the statement as "rather not true", however, in fact remained below 0 for both the score progression as well as the progression in the number of correct answers, signalling an actual decrease in performance compared to the first sound-discrimination test. In this context, the subjects' knowledge of having been part of the trained group seems to clearly influence their judgement of their test performance. The control group's self-evaluation appears more realistic in this sense, even though the mean of subjects having confirmed the statement as "rather true" in fact achieved a slight increase in performance in the second sound-discrimination test. Both the mean of subjects rejecting the statement as "not true" and "rather not true" did show a better performance in the second test, with the graph, however, revealing its peak for the mean of subjects who were less decisive in their answer by selecting the "rather not true" option.

The same effect of over-estimation on the side of the trained group can be seen in the graphs showing the correlation between the subjects' performance progression and their response to the statement of the two tests being equally difficult.[208] The mean of subjects from the trained group who decisively confirmed the statement as "true" in fact showed a notable decrease in their test performance compared to the initial test. Considering the fact that the rejection of the statement comprises both deviation directions, in theory, a level graph at the height of 0 would have been expected. In practice, the graphs representing the control group are clearly closer towards the expected shape than those representing the trained group. Again, the trained group's knowledge of having received a special training seems to have influenced their answers in evaluating their test performances.

207 cf. figures A.3-68 and A.3-69 ibid.
208 cf. figures A.3-70 and A.3-71 ibid.

7 Summary

The aim of the present study was to investigate to what extent adults' perceptive abilities in an unknown foreign language can be enhanced by a non-theory based aural training in music. Music and language are the two methods of conveying meaning by acoustic signals. It was hypothesised that a musical intervention focusing on the discrimination of acoustic signals can improve human sound-discrimination abilities in foreign languages. The increasing interest in the beneficial potential of music on both productive and receptive aspects of language acquisition has been triggered by recent discoveries in neuroscience which provide evidence for cerebral activity during music processing in brain areas earlier believed to exclusively process language. The expected effect on human sound-discrimination abilities in a foreign language could be partially proved by a significant enhancement of the test performance in terms of final scores achieved by the trained group compared to an insignificant enhancement achieved by the control group.

Previous studies have investigated both the receptive strategy of music application for a benefit in the language domain and the productive strategy of active participation in the music. However, a central point of interest in many studies, whether following the one or the other approach, has been the development of listening skills. In previous studies, the time related aspects of music, such as meter, rhythm and tempo have been investigated in context with reading abilities and literacy skills[209] and the space-related aspects of music, such as pitch, melody and harmony, have been examined in context with phonetic, semantic and syntactic processing.[210] In the treatment of dyslexic children, the application of music instruction focused on the time-related aspects of music could be shown to have a positive effect on dyslexic children's reading abilities[211] and rapid timing skills as well as rhythm skills, which were singled out as areas of special difficulty for dyslexic children.[212] The processing of the space-related aspects of music has been shown to bear parallels to the processing of the larger sense units in speech responsible for meaning and structure. In this sense e.g., melody processing has been compared with syntax processing as well as melody production with sentence production. Melodic abilities have also been analysed in context with the ability to use prosodic information as a means of understanding foreign languages in particular and the processing of linguistic intonation in general.[213] When investigating harmonic processing, parallels to the processing of language, especially to the processing of syntactic information, could be shown.[214] The processing of pitch-related information has been of interest in comparison with phonetic processing and with linguistic intonation.[215] Furthermore, music has been applied to test its ability to activate

209 cf. e.g. Overy et al. (2003); Douglas and Willats (1994)
210 cf. e.g. Brown, Martinez and Parsons (2006); Patel (2003), Koelsch et al. (2004); Maess et al. (2001)
211 cf. Douglas and Willats (1994)
212 cf. Overy et al. (2003)
213 cf. Patel and Peretz (1997); Becker (1999); Patel (2003); Brown, Martinez and Parsons (2006)
214 cf. Koelsch et al. (2002); Maess et al. (2001)
215 cf. Patel and Peretz (1997); Zatorre et al. (1992)

semantic-representation areas in the brain.[216] And finally, training in music has been of large interest in the context of memory enhancement, especially in the context of the suggestopedic approach to foreign-language learning, for the benefit of enhancing verbal memory and verbal learning.[217] The plurality and diversity of studies aimed at the investigation of parallels between language and music production, perception, processing and memorising all stress the interconnectivity of strategies and processes involved in the management of both domains. While some shared processes in the perception and production of music and language have already been demonstrated, other seeming parallels still remain unexplained.

Sound discrimination abilities, or auditory discriminative abilities, are in their very general form the competence of distinguishing among acoustic signals. In addition to the separation into different domains of application, sound discrimination abilities can be further subdivided into single abilities. Warren suggests a division into the ability to discriminate loudness, the ability to discriminate phonemes and the ability to discriminate musical sounds.[218] Phoneme-discrimination ability, the sound-discrimination ability in the focus of the present study, is the human competence of distinguishing among isolated speech-sounds important for the formation of larger meaning-carrying entities. This ability is universal at birth but specialises towards an ability to distinguish between language-specifically relevant phonemic contrasts very early in infancy.[219] Theories on the processes involved in speech perception are manifold and comprise for example the motor theory of speech perception, the cohort theory, the trace model of speech recognition and many others.[220] While differing in various aspects, many theories share the idea of the role of phonemic processing in the course of processes involved in speech perception. After an immediate and automatic analysis of the acoustic features of an incoming signal, phonemic processing takes place as a first step of conscious speech processing. This prominent position in the course of speech perception and word recognition underlines the importance of phoneme-discrimination ability for the process of speech perception. Adults' phoneme-discrimination abilities in foreign languages depend on the discrepancy between the phonemic material forming the learner's first language and the set of phonemes relevant for the foreign language to be learned. Success or failure in the discrimination of phonemic differences inexistent in the learner's first language or other previously learned languages depends on the nature of the phonemes, on the time elapsed between the acoustic signals to be distinguished and the amount of practice in discriminating between the non-native phonemes.

The critical age theory for language acquisition, also known as the critical period hypothesis for language learning, assumes an age window, in which language learning has to be initiated in order to be accomplished at all.[221] According to Lenneberg, the edges of this age window are defined by physical immaturity before the age of 2 and by a loss of flexibility for cerebral reorganisation after the age of 12,

216 cf. Koelsch et al. (2004)
217 cf. Ho, Cheung and Chan (2003) ; Brislan (1990); Chan, Ho and Cheung (1998)
218 cf. Warren (1978)
219 cf. e.g. Anderson and Morgan (2003); Werker (1991)
220 cf. Libermann and Cooper (1963); Marslen-Wilson and Welsh (1978); McClelland and Elman (1986)
221 cf. Lenneberg (1967)

by which electro-chemical changes in the brain as well as the lateralisation process for brain functions have been completed. While the loss of the ability to acquire a first language by the onset of puberty has been shown and is not disputed[222], the beginning development of first-language acquisition in the very young infant and the ability to acquire a second or further language after puberty have both been widely discussed, especially in context with adults' non-native phoneme discrimination abilities and production abilities. While it could be shown that a specialisation toward the first language's set of phonemes is already completed in the first year after birth, this specialisation revealed a flexible rather than a fixed end state also for late learners, who could be trained to discriminate among non-native phonemes.[223]

The testing of human sound-discrimination abilities, in particular speech-sound discrimination abilities, dates back as far as 1931 with Travis and Rasmus[224] pioneering the examination of differences in the speech-sound discrimination skills of subjects ranging in age from junior primary school children to adults. Whereas sound-discrimination ability tests generally refer to tests of any kind of acoustical input including the testing of speech-sound, noise and music, the focus in the context of the present study was directed to speech-sound discrimination. In addition to the general testing of human sound-discrimination abilities, which can be subdivided into the testing of subjects' individual progress in sound-discrimination ability over a period of time[225] and the comparison of different test groups' sound-discrimination abilities[226], and the obvious application of sound-discrimination tests in the diagnostics of and research in the domain of hearing impairment[227], tests of this kind have also been carried out to survey possible correlations between sound discrimination abilities and reading abilities[228], pronunciation and articulation abilities[229] and verbal memory[230]. Further studies employing sound-discrimination testing have been e.g. concerned with the preference of information input in either acoustical or visual form over the respective other[231]. Studies and tests on the sound-discrimination in foreign languages are comparatively rare and sound-discrimination in foreign languages unknown to the subjects appears hitherto neglected. This, in addition to the fact that the majority of previous testing methods were developed and designed to match the requirements of very young subjects, necessitated the development of a new speech-sound discrimination test to meet the requirements of the present study.

The test of adults' sound-discrimination abilities in an unknown foreign language developed and applied in the context of the present study consists of two separate online multiple-choice tests, which were carried out at an interval of two weeks. The foreign language examined in this context was Finnish, which is a phonetic language and thus well suited for the present testing purposes, since the

222 cf. Lenneberg (1967), chapter 4 for a wide-spread overview of age of first language onset
223 cf. e.g. Anderson and Morgan (2003); Werker (1991); Wang and Kuhl (2003)
224 Travis and Rasmus (1931)
225 cf. Mansur (1950); Pronovost and Dumbleton (1953); Wepman (1958); Snow and Hoefnagel-Höhle (1979)
226 cf. Templin (1943); Templin (1957); Danhauer, Crawford and Edgerton (1984)
227 cf. Bradley (1972); Finnegan (1974); Bochner et al. (1997)
228 cf. Cabot (1968); Anvari et al. (2002)
229 cf. Travis and Rasmus (1931); Sherman and Geith (1967)
230 cf. Gromko et al. (2009)
231 cf. Camp (1970)

subjects, as novices to the sound of the language, were thus able to match the aural input of heard sounds with the visual input of written characters presented to them in the course of the test. Each test consisted of 62 questions with nine grades of difficulty and eight different question types comprising questions on the number of words heard in a sentence, the identification of a word heard at a specific position in a sentence, the identification of a heard word out of a set of written words, the recognition of the location of a written word in a heard sentence, the identification of a written word out of a set of heard words, the sorting of word orders of heard sentences, the detection of deviations between a heard sentence and its written representation and the identification of a heard sentence out of a set of written sentences. To ensure comparability, the second test consists of the same questions in the same order as those of the first test with different words and phrases of the same level of complexity.

Testing and training methods in the field of musical listening skills appear to differentiate between non- or not-yet-musicians and musicians in their choice and characteristics of applied tasks. Whereas the available methods for aural training in music seem to exclusively direct themselves at musicians and learners of instruments, the so called musicality tests or musical aptitude tests presuppose a not-yet-musician as a potential test taker. In the present study, non-musicians were to receive aural training in music without any reference to music theory and with a strong focus on musical sound discrimination, which necessitated the development of a new training conception comprising discrimination tasks based on unknown music examples in the fields of pitch, tempo, melody, rhythm and harmony at different levels of difficulty executable on a self-study base with answer feedback and fixed timing and omitting the inclusion of music theory and theoretic tasks, instrumental practice and practical tasks. In order to meet all these requirements, the computer-based training program ToSCA (Training of Sound Contrasting Abilities), has been developed and applied. The special focus of ToSCA lies on the training of contrasting, recognition and anticipation of single sounds, sound sequences and sound patterns in the form of music. ToSCA was programmed for fourteen subsequent training units of fifteen minutes daily for a period of two weeks. The single sessions were automatically terminated by the program after fifteen minutes of training and the program remained locked until the following day. In order to achieve the desired teaching effect, all displayed answer options were shaded with red colour for the wrong answers and green colour for the correct answer after an answer choice had been made by the subject. The program covered five different fields of training: pitch, tempo, melody, rhythm and harmony, with each field of training further subdivided into five different levels of difficulty, which could be achieved independently of the respective other fields in order to guarantee a subject-individual training at the trainee's own speed of learning and individual skills. The program was based on six different types of questions aimed at the sound discrimination, recognition and anticipation skills to be trained: the direct comparison between two sounds, the recognition of a given sound from a selection of others, the identification of the one sound from a selection of sounds which differs the most from the first heard sound, the selection of the most fitting sound for the conclusion of an unfinished melody or harmony sequence, the identification of the one sound from a selection of sounds which would not lead an unfinished melody or harmony sequence back to a musically logical ending, and the matching of a heard sound sequence with a suitable graphical representation. The score assignment for questions answered by the subject was programmed to both add points for correct answers and deduct points for wrong answers in order to avoid any possible progress to the next higher level by pure guessing. The level borders were determined after previous testing of the program, according to the training duration and in accordance with the expected performance of the musically untrained subjects.

In the course of the study, 25 subjects constituting a trained group underwent an examination consisting of three phases and 25 further subjects constituting a control group took part in the first and third step of the examination leaving out the interventional phase of the experiment. All 50 test persons were students of non-linguistic subjects at German universities and neither of the test persons had taken part in either instrumental or vocal education or received any other kind of training in music beyond the obligatory music education at school prior to the experiment. The trained group consisted of 11 female and 14 male subjects between 21 and 30 years of age and the control group consisted of 14 female and 11 male subjects between 20 and 33 years of age.

In the first testing phase, the subjects were surveyed on their prior experience with and education in foreign languages and on their music-consumption habits in a questionnaire and subsequently underwent a pre-intervention examination on sound discrimination and word recognition in Finnish as described above. In the second testing phase, the trained subjects were granted two weeks time in order to carry out the self-study based music-training program ToSCA introduced above while the control subjects had two weeks time without any testing. The third testing phase consisted of a second language test equivalent to the pre-intervention examination referred to above and a self-evaluation survey on the subjects' impressions of their own achievements in both sound-discrimination tests.

The main hypothesis of the present study was focused on the expectation of stronger increased sound-discrimination test results achieved by the trained group in contrast to the performance increase achieved by the control group, which proved true for the improvement in terms of final score. The mean final scores achieved by the trained group were significantly better in the second sound-discrimination test, whereas the mean final scores achieved by the control group improved only insignificantly. An improvement for both groups was predicted due to an expected effect of familiarisation with the test method and test language and thus does not interfere with the hypothesis. A significant increase in the number of correct answers, however, could not be shown for either the control group or the trained group. Furthermore, the difference between the control group's performance enhancement and the trained groups enhancement, in the end, failed to prove significant. Even though the trends towards a potential influence of ToSCA on the results achieved in the post-intervention sound-discrimination test were obvious, the expected effect could not be shown with significant differences compared to the results achieved by the control group. This could finally be attributed to a too short time of intervention as well as to an insufficient number of participants.

A detailed analysis of the influence of the single training fields of ToSCA on the single sound-discrimination test categories revealed a strong impact on subjects' performance enhancement in their ability to locate a word in a sentence. This ability was shown to depend on subjects' performance in almost all ToSCA training categories except for melody training. While a relationship with the time-related categories, i.e. rhythm and tempo, was expected, the additional relation with the space-related categories of pitch and harmony was a surprise. Furthermore, the initially hypothesised positive effect of a good performance in the training field of tempo on the ability to identify the number of words in a sentence could be confirmed by the results. Other expected correlations between the performance in the time-related training fields of ToSCA and those sound-discrimination test questions focused on larger entities, i.e. sentences, as well as further expected relationships between the space-related training fields of ToSCA and the phoneme-focused sound-discrimination test questions could not be shown.

The hypothesised dependence of the subjects' test performances on their previous language-learning and application experience revealed some interesting correlations. Contrary to expectation, a dependency of the first sound-discrimination test results on subjects' prior language-learning could not be shown. However, the performance enhancement from the first to the second sound-discrimination test proved strongly dependent on the number of foreign languages used in every-day life, which was an expected dependency.

The expected differences in ToSCA training achievement for subjects with different music-type preferences proved true in terms of subjects with an affinity for rhythm-focused types of music achieving notably better results in the rhythm-training category than other subjects and subjects with an affinity for melody-focused types of music achieving considerably better in the melody-training category than other subjects. The further hypothesised effects of an affinity towards melody-focused types of music on the results in pitch training and of an affinity towards rhythm-focused types of music on the results in tempo training could not be shown. As expected, subjects with a preference for multi-focal types of music performed significantly better in the training category of harmony as well as in the final ToSCA training result. In a further study, it may be interesting to compare the results of subjects with a preference for types of music with the same musical focus.

Training achievement with ToSCA was furthermore expected to depend on subjects' usual degree of participation in the music they listen to with no participation correlating with lower achievement, the invention of new melodies while singing along correlating with a high performance in melody training and the invention of new rhythms while tapping or clapping along correlating with a high result in rhythm training. These correlations could not be shown exactly as expected. However, the expected results for the subjects' participation by singing could be found in favour of the harmony-training category. This may seem self-explanatory in retrospect since the invention of a new melody matching the music naturally requires a mental conception of and feeling for the harmonic procedure of the respective piece of music.

Furthermore, a positive effect of a high number of hours spent on actively listening to music per day on the subjects' performance in the training with ToSCA was expected and could be shown for the percentage of correct answers, which proved significantly higher for every further hour of active music listening.

The number of languages currently used by the subjects was hypothesised to correlate with their test performance and could be shown for the total performance progression from the first to the second sound-discrimination test. As hypothesised, the more languages currently used by the subject, the higher the subjects' receptivity towards a new language. Beneficial effects could especially be shown for questions focusing on the sentence level of language.

The expected trend in the context of self-evaluation of the trained group being more likely to select the extreme answer options of "true" or "not true" than the control group proved true for almost all statements. Also the hypothesis on the trained group's subjects classifying their performance in the second sound-discrimination test as better than in the first test could be verified. The expected correspondence of the subjects' stating their immediate accustomisation to the sound of the new language and a good performance in the first sound-discrimination test already only proved true for the trained group. The subjects' response to the statements directly comparing the two sound discrimination tests could only partially show the expected correlation with their actual performance and performance progression. Whereas the statement of the first test being experienced as more difficult than the second test did reveal a correlation with the subjects' actual performance, there was no correlation between the opposite statement of the second sound-discrimination test being experienced as more difficult than the first one and the subjects' actual performance. The trained group's performance estimation could finally reveal a stronger conviction of having performed better in the second as opposed to the first sound-discrimination test than the control group's performance estimation.

Future studies on the here only partially provable influence of training in the discrimination of musical sounds on linguistic sound-discrimination abilities should include more subjects and longer training periods while reducing the multitude of possible impacts. Subjects in this study, while being largely homogeneous in their inexperience in music training, age, education level and inexperience in linguistic studies, were still diverse in their level of experience with foreign language learning, their amount of foreign-language usage and many other aspects. It may be interesting to further reduce these diversities in order to achieve more precise results. Furthermore, other foreign languages should be used for further testing. Speech sounds, however, just as in the present study, should not be singled out of their natural syntactic contexts in order to achieve a test situation which is based on linguistically natural contexts as far as possible without constituting a clinically reduced speech event.

Bibliography

A

Anderson, Jennifer L.; Morgan, J. L. (2003). A Statistical Basis for Speech Sound Discrimination. In *Language and Speech*. 46(2-3). (155-182).

Anvari, Sima H. et al. (2002). Relations among musical skills, phonological processing, and early reading ability in preschool children. In *Journal of Experimental Child Psychology*. 83(2). (111-130).

Appelbaum, Irene (1996). The Lack of Invariance Problem and the Goal of Speech Perception. In *International Conference on Spoken Language Processing*. 96. (1541-1544).

B

Bancrof, W. Jane (1999). *Suggestopedia and Language Acquisition: Variations on a Theme*. Amsterdam: Gordon and Breach.

Baroni, Mario (1991). Interrelationships between verbal and musical grammars. In Sundberg, Johan; Nord, L., Carlson, R. (eds.) *Music, Language, Speech and Brain*. Houndmills, Basingstoke: Macmillan.

Barwick, Julia et al. (1989). Relations between reading and musical abilities. In *British Journal of Educational Psychology*. 59. (253-257).

Becker, Monika (1999). *Ist am Anfang wirklich nur das Wort? Zur Funktion der Prosodie im Fremdsprachenlernen.* Aachen: Shaker Verlag.

Bellis, Teri J. (1997). *Assessment and Management of Central Auditory Processing Disorders in the Educational Setting. From Science to Practice*. London: Singular Publishing Group.

Bendig, Volker (1999). *Elementare Gehörbildung. Von den Anfängen bis zur Aufnahmeprüfung an einer wissenschaftlichen Hochschule*. Essen: Die Blaue Eule.

Bentley, Arnold (1966). *Measures of Musical Abilities*. London: George G. Harrap & Co. Ltd.

Besson, Mireille; Schön, Daniele (2003). Comparison between Language and Music. In Peretz, Isabelle; Zatorre, R. J. (eds.) *The Cognitive Neuroscience of Music*. New York: Oxford University Press.

Best, Catherine T. (1993). Emergence of Language-Specific Constraints in Perception of Non-Native Speech: A Window on Early Phonological Development. In Boysson-Bardies, Bénédicte de; Schonen, S. de (eds.) *Developmental Neurocognition: Speech and Face Processing in the First Year of Life*. New York: Kluwer.

Best, Catherine T. (1995). Learning to Perceive the Sound Pattern of English. In Rovee-Collier, Carolin; Lipsitt, L. P. (eds.) *Advances in Infancy Research*. Norwood, New Jersey: Ablex.

Best, Catherine T. (1999). Development of Language-Specific Influences on Speech Perception and Production in Pre-Verbal Infancy. In *International Congress of Phonetic Sciences*. 99. (1261-1264).

Bharucha, Jamshed J. (1991). Cognitive and brain mechanisms in perceptual learning. In Sundberg, Johan; Nord, L.; Carlson, R. (eds.) *Music, Language, Speech and Brain*. Houndmills, Basingstoke: Macmillan.

Bialystok, Ellen; Hakuta, Kenji (1999). Confounded Age: Linguistic and Cognitive Factors in Age Differences for Second Language Acquisition. In Birdsong, David (ed.) *Second Language Acquisition and the Critical Period Hypothesis*. Mahwah, New Jersey and London: Lawrence Erlbaum Associates.

Birdsong, David (ed.) (1999). *Second Language Acquisition and the Critical Period Hypothesis*. Mahwah, New Jersey and London: Lawrence Erlbaum Associates.

Birkenshaw-Fleming, Lois (1990). Music and Language Development. In Dobbs, Jack (ed.) *Music Education: Facing the Future*. Rading: International Society for Music Education.

Bochner, Joseph et al. (1997). A computerized adaptive testing system for speech discrimination measurement: The Speech Sound Pattern Discrimination Test. In *Journal of the Acoustical Society of America*. 101(4). (2289-2298).

Bosch, Laura; Sebastián-Gallés, N. (2005). Developmental Changes in the Discrimination of Vowel Contrasts in Bilingual Infants. In Cohen, James et al. (eds.) *Proceedings of the 4th International Symposium on Bilingualism*. (354-361). Somerville: Cascadilla Press.

Boysson-Bardies, Bénédicte de; Schonen, S. de (eds.) (1993). *Developmental Neurocognition: Speech and Face Processing in the First Year of Life*. New York: Kluwer.

Bradley, Betty H. (1972). Responses of retardates to three auditory discrimination tests. In *International Journal of Disability, Development and Education*. 19(1). (22-27).

Bradshaw, John L. (1985). Funktionseinteilung im Gehirn. In Bruhn, Herbert; Oerter, R.; Rösing, H. (eds.) *Musikpsychologie. Ein Handbuch in Schlüsselbegriffen*. München; Wien; Baltimore: Urban & Schwarzenberg.

Brislan, Patrick S. (1990). Suggestopedic Communication – Parallels between Foreign Language Instruction and Music Education. In Dobbs, Jack (ed.) *Music Education: Facing the Future*. Reading: ISME.

Brown, Roger (1981). Music and Language. In Music Educators National Conference. *Report of the Ann Arbor Symposium on the Applications of Psychology to the Teaching and Learning of Music*. (233-264).

Brown, Steven; Martinez, M. J.; Parsons, L. M. (2006). Music and language side by side in the brain: a PET study of the generation of melodies and sentences. In *European Journal of Neuroscience*. 23. (2791-2803).

Brunner, Monika; Dierks, A.; Seibert, A. (2005). *Heidelberger Lautdifferenzierungstest. H-LAD. 2. erweiterte Auflage mit Normwerten für die Klassen 1, 2, 3 und 4*. Wertingen: Westra Elektroakustik.

C

Cabot, Raymond (1968). *The construction and validation of the Michigan auditory discrimination test*. PhD thesis. University of Michigan.

Camp, Sarah S. van (1970). *An auditory and visual discrimination test for kindergarten and first grade children. A new approach*. PhD thesis. University of Massachusetts.

Campbell, Don G. (2001). *The Mozart effect: tapping the power of music to heal the body, strengthen the mind, and unlock the creative spirit*. London: Hodder & Stoughton.

Carroll, John B. (1993). *Human cognitive abilities. A survey of factor-analytic studies*. New York: Cambridge University Press.

Carterette, Edward C.; Friedman, M. C. (eds.) (1978). *Handbook of Perception. Volume X. Perceptual Ecology*. New York, San Francisco and London: Academic Press.

Chan, Agnes S.; Ho, Y.; Cheung, M. (1998). Music training improves verbal memory. In *Nature*. 396. (128).

Cohen, Antonie (1975). Measuring Intelligibility in Foreign-Language Learning. In Essen, Arnold J. van; Menting, J. P. (eds.) *The Context of Foreign-Language Learning*. (5-17). Assen: Van Gorcum & Comp B.V.

Cohen, Antonie; Nooteboom, S. G. (eds.) (1975). *Structure and Process in Speech Perception*. (16-34). Berlin; Heidelberg: Springer-Verlag.

Colwell, Richard; Richardson, C. (eds.) (2002). *The New Handbook of Research on Music Teaching and Learning: A Project of the Music Educators National Conference*. Oxford: Oxford University Press.

Coren, Stanley; Ward, L. M.; Enns, J. T. (2004). *Sensation and Perception*. Sixth Edition. Hoboken: John Wiley & Sons.

Cranmer, David; Laroy, C. (1992). *Musical Openings: Using Music in the Language Classroom*. Harlow: Longman.

Cross, Ian; Howell, P.; West, R. (1985). Structural Relationships in the Perception of Musical Pitch. In Howell, Peter (ed.) *Musical Structure and Cognition*. London: Academic Press.

D

Danhauer, Jeffrey L.; Crawford, S.; Edgerton, B. J. (1984). English, Spanish, and Bilingual Speakers' Performance on a Nonsense Syllable Test (NST) of Speech Sound Discrimination. In *Journal of Speech and Hearing Disorders*. 49. (164-184).

Dirven, René (1977). Aspekte der Hörverstehensfertigkeit. In Dirven, René (ed.) *Hörverständnis im Fremdsprachenunterricht*. (1-13). Kronberg: Scriptor Verlag.

Dobbs, Jack (ed.) (1990). *Music Education: Facing the Future*. Reading: International Society for Music Education.

Douglas, Sheila; Willats, P. (1994). The relationship between musical ability and literacy skills. In *Journal of Research in Reading*. 17(2). (99-107).

E

Ehrenfels, Christian von (1988). The Presentation of a Melody. The Thesis of Gestalt Qualities. In Smith, Barry (ed.) *Foundations of Gestalt Theory*. (82-116). München and Wien: Philosophia Verlag.

F

Finnegan, Denis E. (1974). Speech Sound Discrimination Skills of Seven- and Eight-Year-Old Cleft Palate Males. In *Cleft Palate Journal*. 11(2). (111-122).

Fried, Lilian (1980). *Lautunterscheidungstest für Vorschulkinder (4-7 Jahre). LUT*. Weinheim: Beltz Verlag.

Fox, John (2002). *An R and S-Plus Companion to Applied Regression*. Thousand Oaks: Sage.

Füller, Klaus (1974). *Standardisierte Musiktests*. Frankfurt am Main: Verlag Moritz Diesterweg.

G

Giauque, Gerlad S. (1985). *Foreign Language Acquisition and the Study of Music*. Northern Arizona University: Microfiche.

Goldberg, Merryl; Scott-Kassner, Carol (2002). Teaching Other Subjects through Music. In Colwell, Richard; Richardson, C. (eds.) (2002) *The New Handbook of Research on Music Teaching and Learning: A Project of the Music Educators National Conference*. Oxford: Oxford University Press.

Gordon-Brannan, Mary E.; Weiss, C. E. (2007). *Clinical Management of Articulatory and Phonologic Disorders*. Third Edition. Baltimore; Philadelphia: Lippincott Williams & Wilkins.

Griffiths, Timothy D. (2003). The neural processing of complex sounds. In Peretz, Isabelle; Zatorre, R. J. (eds.) *The Cognitive Neuroscience of Music*. New York: Oxford University Press.

Gromko, Joyce E. (2005). The Effect of Music Instruction on Phonemic Awareness in Beginning Readers. In *Journal of Research in Music Education*. 53(3). (199-209).

Gromko, Joyce E. et al. (2009). Effects of Temporal Sequencing and Auditory Discrimination on Children's Memory Patterns for Tones, Numbers, and Nonsense Words. In *Journal of Research in Music Eduction*. 57(2). (140-151).

Gruhn, Wilfried; Rauscher, Frances (2002). The Neurobiology of Music Cognition and Learning. In Colwell, Richard; Richardson, C. (eds.) *The New Handbook of Research on Music Teaching and Learning: A Project of the Music Educators National Conference*. Oxford: Oxford University Press.

H

Ho, Yim-Chi; Cheung, M.; Chan, A. S. (2003). Music Training Improves Verbal but Not Visual Memory: Cross-Sectional and Longitudinal Explorations in Children. In *Neuropsychology*. 17(3). (439-450).

Holahan, John M.; Saunders, T. C. (2000). Tonal Cognition in Pattern Discrimination: Evidence from Three Populations. In *Journal of Research in Music Education*. 48(2). (162-177).

Howell, Peter (ed.) (1985). *Musical Structure and Cognition*. London: Academic Press.

J

Johnson, Jacqueline S.; Newport, Elissa L. (1989). Critical Period Effects in Second Language Learning: The Influence of Maturational State on the Acquisition of English as a Second Language. In *Cognitive Psychology*. 21. (60-99).

Jusczyk, Peter W.; Luce, P. A. (2002). Speech Perception and Spoken Word Recognition: Past and Present. In *Ear & Hearing*. 23(2). (2-40).

K

Kaiser, Ulrich (1998). *Gehörbildung. Satzlehre. Improvisation. Höranalyse. Ein Lehrgang mit historischen Beispielen*. Kassel: Bärenreiter.

Koelsch, Stefan et al. (2002). Bach Speaks: A Cortical "Language-Network" Serves the Processing of Music. In *NeuroImage*. 17. (956-966).

Koelsch, Stefan et al. (2004). Music, language and meaning: brain signatures of semantic processing. In *Nature Neuroscience*. 7(3). (302-307).

Krumhansl, Carol L.; Toiviainen, P. (2003). Tonal Cognition. In Peretz, Isabelle; Zatorre, R. J. (eds.) *The Cognitive Neuroscience of Music*. New York: Oxford University Press.

Kühn, Clemens (1983). *Gehörbildung im Selbststudium*. Kassel: Bärenreiter.

L

Lamb, Susannah J.; Gregory, A. H. (1993). The relationship between music and reading in beginning readers. In *Educational Psychology*. 13(1). (19-26).

Lee, Christopher S. (1995). The Rhythmic Interpretation of Simple Musical Sequences: Towards a Perceptual Model. In Howell, Peter (ed.) *Musical Structure and Cognition*. London: Academic Press.

Lenneberg, Eric H. (1967). *Biological Foundations of Language*. Malabar, Florida: Robert E. Krieger Publishing Company.

Liberman, Alvin M.; Cooper, F. S. (1963). A Motor Theory of Speech Perception. In *Proceedings of the Speech Communication Seminar*. Stockholm: Royal Institute of Technology.

Liljencrants, Johan (1991). Analogies in the production of speech and music. In Sundberg, Johan; Nord, L., Carlson, R. (eds.) *Music, Language, Speech and Brain*. Houndmills, Basingstoke: Macmillan.

M

Mackamul, Roland (1969). *Lehrbuch der Gehörbildung. Band 1. Elementare Gehörbildung*. Kassel: Bärenreiter.

Maess, Burkhard et al. (2001). Musical syntax is processed in Broca's area: an MEG study. In *Nature Neuroscience*. 4(5). (540-545).

Mansur, R. W. (1950). *The construction of a picture test for speech sound discrimination*. Master of Education thesis. Boston University.

Marslen-Wison, William D.; Welsh, A. (1978). Processing Interactions and Lexical Access during Word Recognition in Continuous Speech. In *Cognitive Psychology*. 10. (29-63).

McCarthy, William G. (1985). Promoting language development through music. In *Academic Therapy*. 21(2). (237-242).

McClelland, James L.; Elman, J. L. (1986). The TRACE Model of Speech Perception. In *Cognitive Psychology*. 18. (1-86).

Merleau-Ponty, Maurice (1981). Speech-Sound Discrimination. In Peterson, H. A.; Marquardt, T. P. (eds.) *Appraisal and diagnosis of speech and language disorders*. Englewood Cliffs: Prentice-Hall.

Metcalfe, Jean V. C. (1962). *An Investigation into Certain Aspects of Speech Sound Discrimination in Children*. PhD Dissertation, Stanford University.

Moskovsky, Christo (2002). The Critical Period Hypothesis Revisited. In Allen, Cynthia (ed.) *Proceedings of the 2001 Conference of the Australian Linguistic Society*. http://www.als.asn.au.

Moyer, Alene (2004). *Age, Accent and Experience in Second Language Acquisition*. Clevedon, Buffalo, Toronto, Sydney: Multilingual Matters Ltd.

Musicians-place.de (2008). *Kurse für Harmonielehre, Rhythmik und Gehörbildung*. Online: http://www.musicians-place.de/ (29.11.2008)

musikwissenschaften.de (2008). *Musik lernen – interaktiv und spielerisch*. Online: http://www.musikwissenschaften.de/ (29.11.2008)

N

Niemeyer, Wilhelm (1970). *Bremer Lautdiskriminationstest*. Bremen: Verlag Paul Herbig.

O

Overy, Katie et al. (2003). Dyslexia and Music: Measuring Musical Timing Skills. In *Dyslexia*. 9. (18-36).

P

Pallasmaa, Juhani (1990). Integrating Art into General Education. Art, Knowledge and Reality: on the cultural significance of art. In Dobbs, Jack (ed.) *Music Education: Facing the Future*. Reading: International Society for Music Education.

Pantev, Christo et al. (2003). Representational cortex in musicians. In Peretz, Isabelle; Zatorre, R. J. (eds.) *The Cognitive Neuroscience of Music*. New York: Oxford University Press.

Pascual-Leone, Alvaro (2003). The brain that makes music and is changed by it. In Peretz, Isabelle; Zatorre, R. J. (eds.) *The Cognitive Neuroscience of Music*. New York: Oxford University Press.

Parsons, Lawrence M. (2003). Exploring the functional neuroanatomy of music performance, perception, and comprehension. In Peretz, Isabelle; Zatorre, R. J. (eds.) *The Cognitive Neuroscience of Music*. New York: Oxford University Press.

Patel, Aniruddh D.; Peretz, I. (1997). Is music autonomous from language? A neuropsychological appraisal. In Deliège, Irène; Sloboda, J. (eds.) *Perception and Cognition of Music*. East Sussex: Psychology Press.

Patel, Aniruddh D. (2003). Language, music, syntax and the brain. In *Nature Neuroscience*. 6(7). (674-681).

Peiyuan, Li; Yuan R. (1979). *Grundkurs der chinesischen Sprache*. Band 1. Beijing: Sinolingua.

Peretz, Isabelle (2003). Brain Specialisation for Music: New Evidence from Congenital Amusia. In Peretz, Isabelle; Zatorre, R. J. (eds.) *The Cognitive Neuroscience of Music*. New York: Oxford University Press.

Peretz, Isabelle; Zatorre, R. J. (eds.) (2003). *The Cognitive Neuroscience of Music*. New York: Oxford University Press.

Pisoni, David B.; Sawusch, J. R. (1975). Some Stages of Processing in Speech Perception. In Cohen, Antonie; Nooteboom, S. G. (eds.) *Structure and Process in Speech Perception*. (16-34). Berlin; Heidelberg: Springer-Verlag.

Pronovost, Wilbert; Dumbleton, C. (1953). A Picture-Type Speech Sound Discrimination Test. In *Journal of Speech and Hearing Disorders*. 18(3). (258-266).

Q

Quistorp, Monika (1970). *Die Gehörbildung. Das Kernfach musikalischer Erziehung*. Wiesbaden: Breitkopf & Härtel.

R

Rauschecker, Josef P. (2003). Functional organization and plasticity of auditory cortex. In Peretz, Isabelle; Zatorre, R. J. (eds.) *The Cognitive Neuroscience of Music*. New York: Oxford University Press.

Repp, Bruno Hermann (1991). Some cognitive and perceptual aspects of speech and music. In Sundberg, Johan; Nord, L.; Carlson, R. (eds.) *Music, Language, Speech and Brain*. Houndmills, Basingstoke: Macmillan.

Rising Software (2003). *Auralia. Complete Ear Training for All Musicians*. Fairfield, Victoria : Rising Software.

Rovee-Collier, Carolin; Lipsitt, L. P. (eds.) (1995). *Advances in Infancy Research*. Norwood, New Jersey: Ablex.

S

Saffran, Jenny R. et al. (1999). Statistical learning of tone sequences by human infants and adults. In *Cognition*. 70. (27-52).

Samson, Séverine; Ehrlé, Nathalie (2003). Cerebral substrates of musical imagery. In Peretz, Isabelle; Zatorre, R. J. (eds.) *The Cognitive Neuroscience of Music*. New York: Oxford University Press.

Seashore, Carl Emil (1960). *Measures of Musical Talent*. Revised Edition. New York: Psychological Corporation.

Schellenberg, E. Glenn (2003). Does exposure to music have beneficial side effects? In Peretz, Isabelle; Zatorre, R. J. (eds.) *The Cognitive Neuroscience of Music*. New York: Oxford University Press.

Schlaug, Gottfried (2003). The brain of musicians. In Peretz, Isabelle; Zatorre, R. J. (eds.) *The Cognitive Neuroscience of Music*. New York: Oxford University Press.

Schlaug, Gottfried et al. (1995). Increased Corpus Callosum Size in Musicians. In *Neuropsychologia*. 33(8). (1047-1055).

Sherman, Dorothy; Geith, A. (1967). Speech Sound Discrimination and Articulation Skill. In *Journal of Speech and Hearing Research*. 10. (277-280).

Singleton, David (1989). *Language Acquisition: The Age Factor*. Clevedon and Philadelphia: Multilingual Matters Ltd.

Snow, Catherine E.; Hoefnagel-Höhle, M. (1979). Individual differences in second-language ability: A factor-analytic study. In *Language and Speech*. 22(2). (151-162).

Stewart, Lauren et al. (2003). Brain changes after learning to read and play music. In *NeuroImage*. 20(1). (71-83).

Stewart, Lauren; Walsh, V.; Frith, U. (2004). Reading music modifies spatial mapping in pianists. In *Perception and Psychophysics*. 66(2). (183-195).

Strickland, Susan J. (2002). Music and the Brain in Childhood Development. In *Childhood Education*. 2002. (100-103).

Sundberg, Johan; Lindblom, B. (1976). Generative theories in language and music descriptions. In *Cognition*. 4. (99-122).

Sundberg, Johan (1991). Summary. In Sundberg, Johan; Nord, L., Carlson, R. (eds.) *Music, Language, Speech and Brain*. Houndmills, Basingstoke: Macmillan.

T

Templin, Mildred C. (1943). A Study of sound discrimination ability of elementary school pupils. In *Journal of Speech Disorders*. 8. (172-132).

Templin, Mildred C. (1957). *Certain Language Skills in Children. Their Development and Interrelationships*. Minneapolis: University of Minnesota Press.

Tervaniemi, Mari (2003). Musical sound processing: EEG and MEG evidence. In Peretz, Isabelle; Zatorre, R. J. (eds.) *The Cognitive Neuroscience of Music*. New York: Oxford University Press.

Thomas, Roswitha (1990). Der Begriff der Gestalt in der Musik und der Psychologie. In Frohne-Hagemann, Isabelle (ed.), *Musik und Gestalt. Klinische Musiktherapie als integrative Psychotherapie*. (17-36). Paderborn: Junfermann Verlag.

Tillmann, Barbara; Bharucha, Jamshed J., Bigand, E. (2003). Learning and perceiving musical structures: further insight from artificial neural networks. In Peretz, Isabelle; Zatorre, R. J. (eds.) *The Cognitive Neuroscience of Music*. New York: Oxford University Press.

Travis, Lee E.; Rasmus, B. (1931). The Speech Sound Discrimination Ability of Cases with Functional Disorders of Articulation. In *The Quarterly Journal of Speech.* 17. (217-226).

V

Venables, William N. & Ripley, R. D. (2002). *Modern Applied Statistics with S.* Fourth edition. New York: Springer.

W

Wang, Yue; Kuhl, P. K. (2003). Evaluating the "Critical Period" Hypothesis: Perceptual Learning of Mandarin Tones in American Adults and American Children at 6, 10 and 14 Years of Age. In *International Congress of Phonetic Sciences.* 2003. (1537-1540).

Warren, David H. (1978). Perception by the Blind. In Carterette, Edward C.; Friedman, M. C. (eds.) *Handbook of Perception. Volume X. Perceptual Ecology.* New York, San Francisco and London: Academic Press.

Watkins, Anthony J.; Dyson, M. C. (1985). On the Perceptual Organisation of Tone Sequences and Melodies. In Howell, Peter (ed.) *Musical Structure and Cognition.* London: Academic Press.

Wepman, Joseph M. (1958). *Auditory Discrimination Test.* Chicago: Joseph M. Wepman.

Werker, Janet (1991). The Ontogeny of Speech Perception. In Mattingly, Ignatius G.; Studdert-Kennedy, M. (eds.) *Modularity and the Motor Theory of Speech Perception.* (91-109). Hillsdale: Lawrence Erlbaum Associates.

Werker, Janet; Logan, J. (1985). Cross-Language Evidence for Three Factors in Speech Perception. In *Perception and Psychophysics.* 37. (35-44).

Wertheimer, Max (1969). Laws of Organization in Perceptual Forms. In Ellis, Willis D. (ed.), A *Source Book of Gestalt Psychology.* (71-88). London: Routledge & Kegan Paul Ltd.

Whitaker, Nancy (1994). Whole Language and Music Education. In *Music Educators Journal.* 81(1). (24-28).

Williams, David B. (1981). Music Information Processing and Memory. In Music Educators National Conference. *Report of the Ann Arbor Symposium on the Applications of Psychology to the Teaching and Learning of Music.* (87-93).

Z

Zatorre, Robert J. et al. (1992). Lateralization of Phonetic and Pitch Discrimination in Speech Processing. In *Science.* 256. (846- 849).

Appendix A Evaluation Graphics

Appendix A.1 Boxplots and Barplots on Scores Achieved and the Number of Correct Answers Given in the Sound-Discrimination Tests

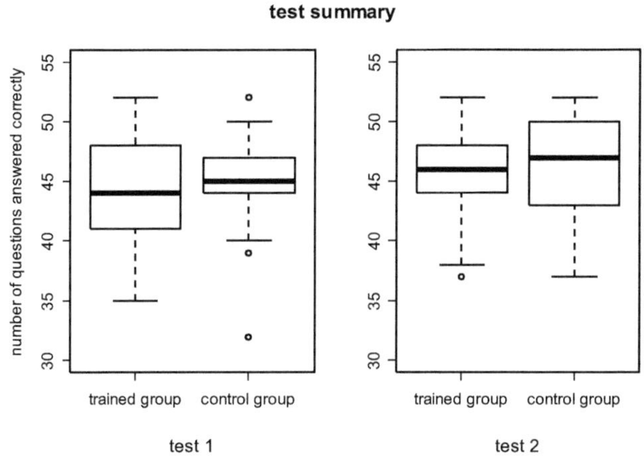

figure A.1-18: boxplots on the number of correct answers given in tests 1 and 2 by the two groups

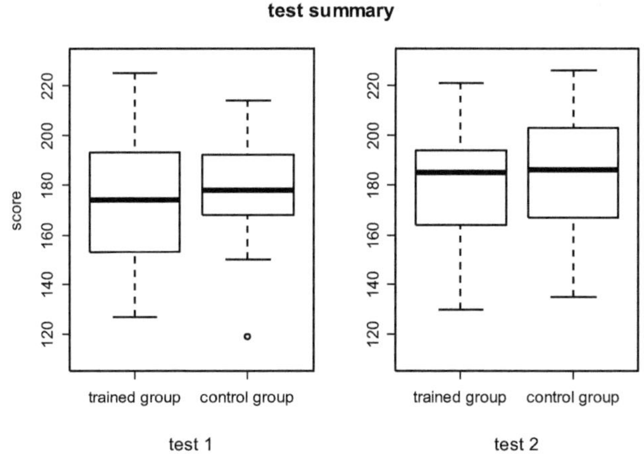

figure A.1-19: boxplots on the scores achieved in tests 1 and 2 by the two groups

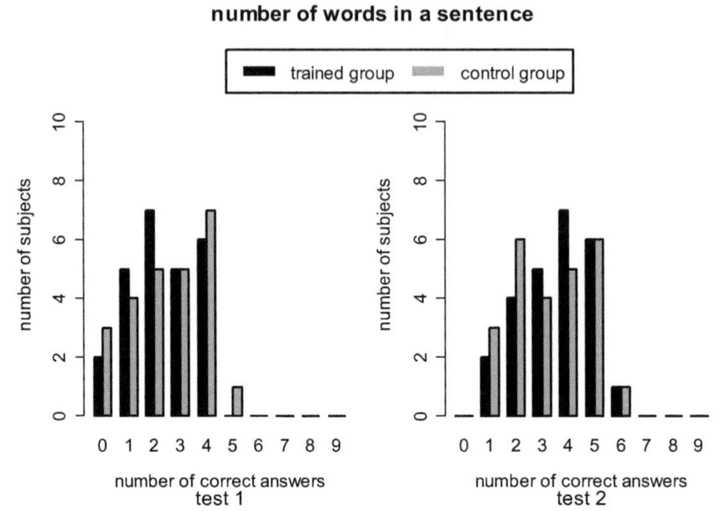

figure A.1-20: barplots on the number of category-one questions answered correctly in tests 1 and 2 by the two groups

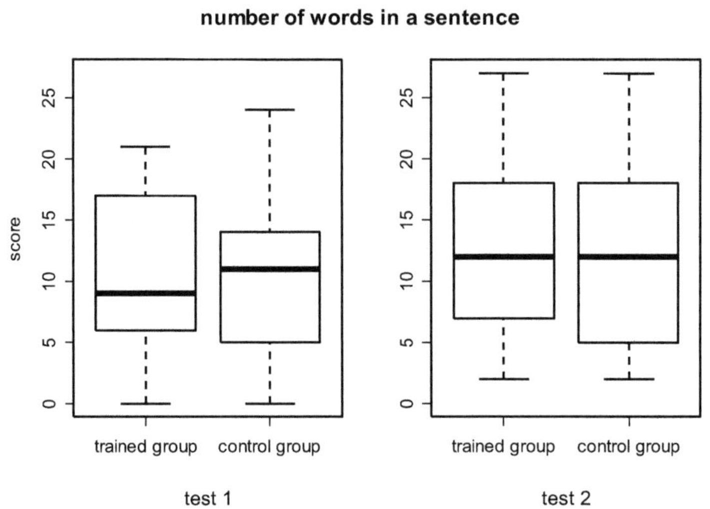

figure A.1-21: boxplots on the scores achieved in question category one in tests 1 and 2 by the two groups

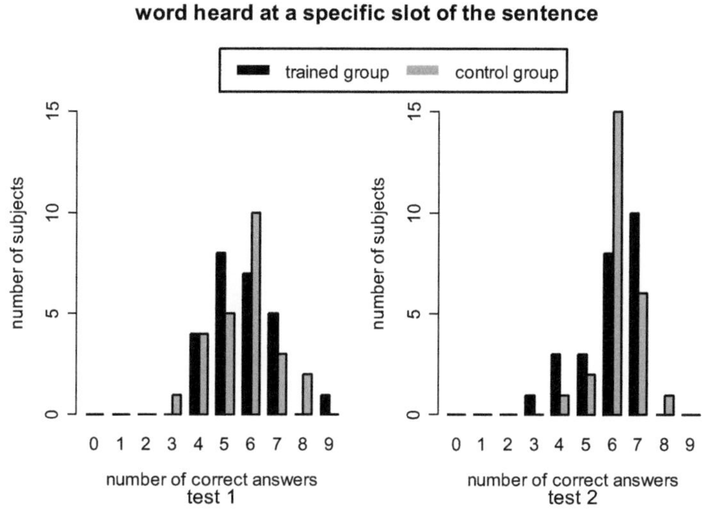

figure A.1-22: barplots on the number of category-two questions answered correctly in tests 1 and 2 by the two groups

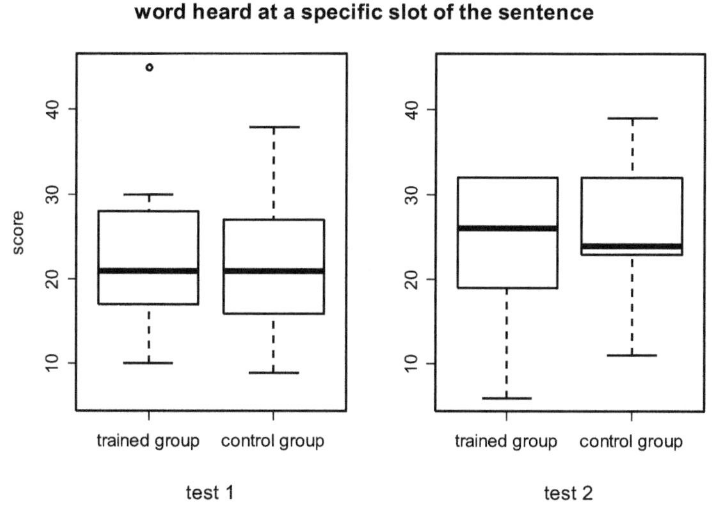

figure A.1-23: boxplots on the scores achieved in question category two in tests 1 and 2 by the two groups

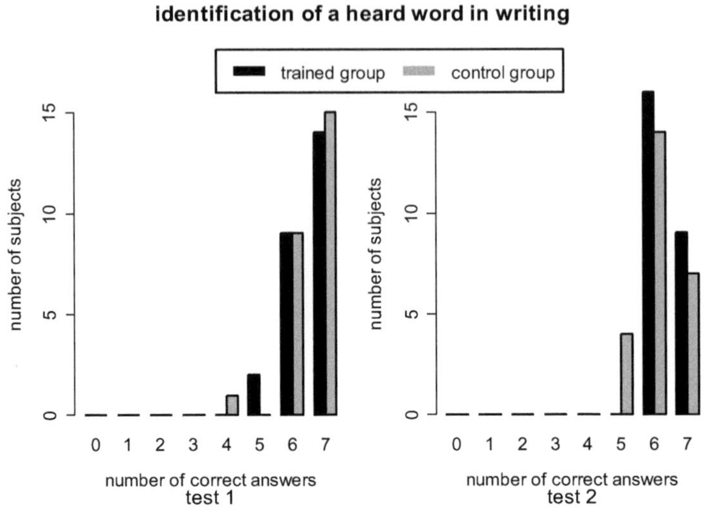

figure A.1-24: barplots on the number of category-three questions answered correctly in tests 1 and 2 by the two groups

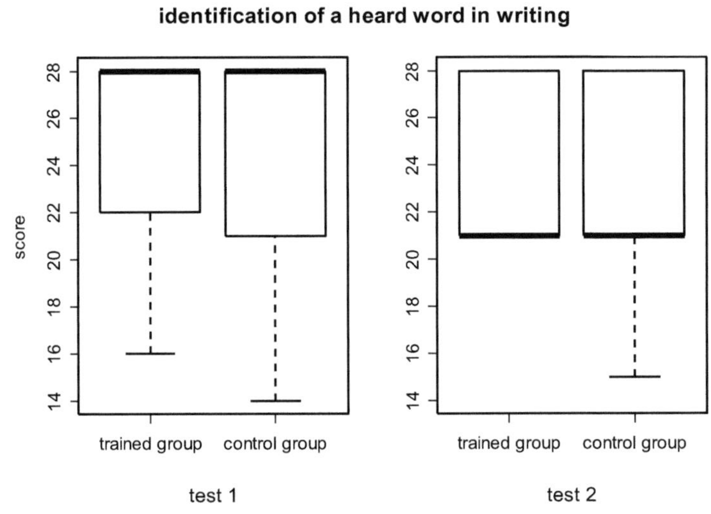

figure A.1-25: boxplots on the scores achieved in question category three in tests 1 and 2 by the two groups

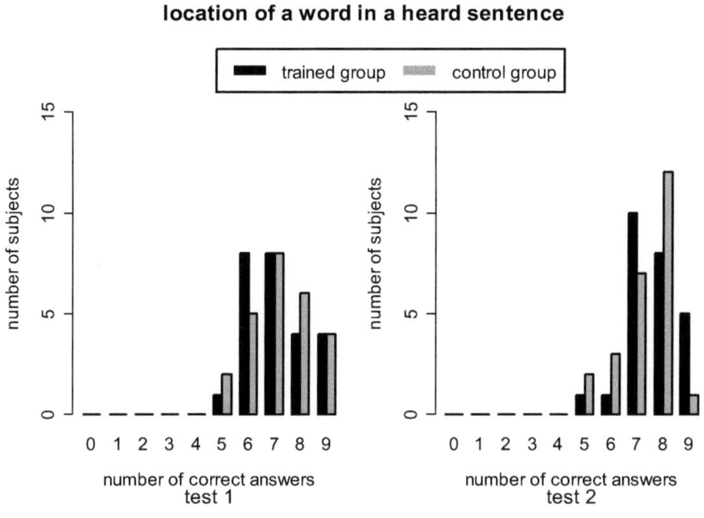

figure A.1-26: barplots on the number of category-four questions answered correctly in tests 1 and 2 by the two groups

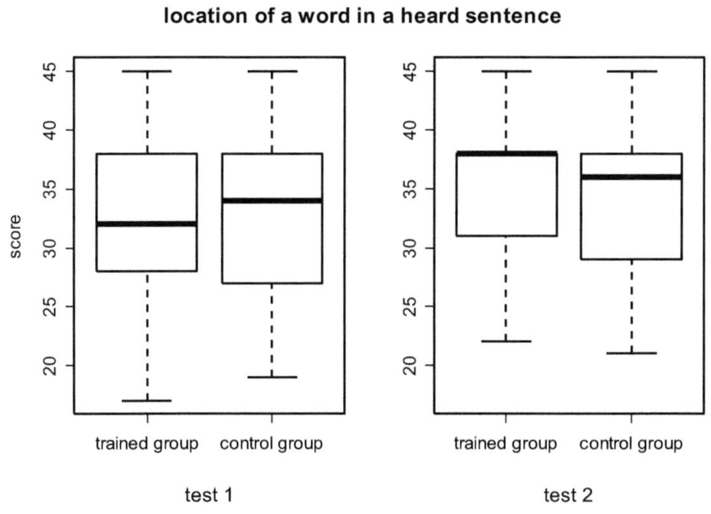

figure A.1-27: boxplots on the scores achieved in question category four in tests 1 and 2 by the two groups

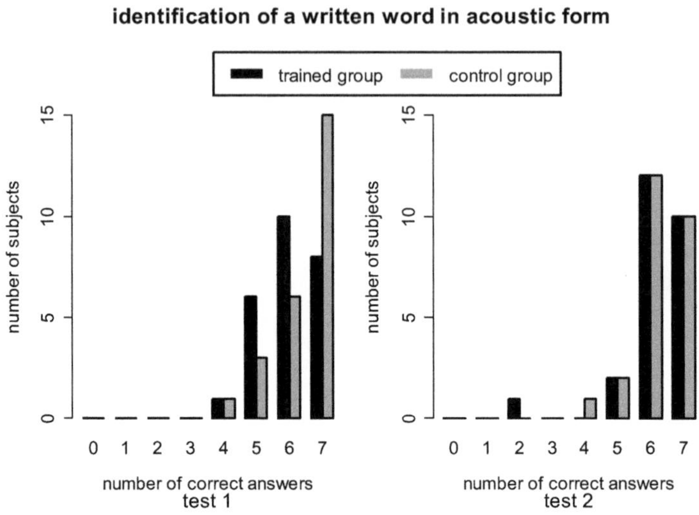

figure A.1-28: barplots on the number of category-five questions answered correctly in tests 1 and 2 by the two groups

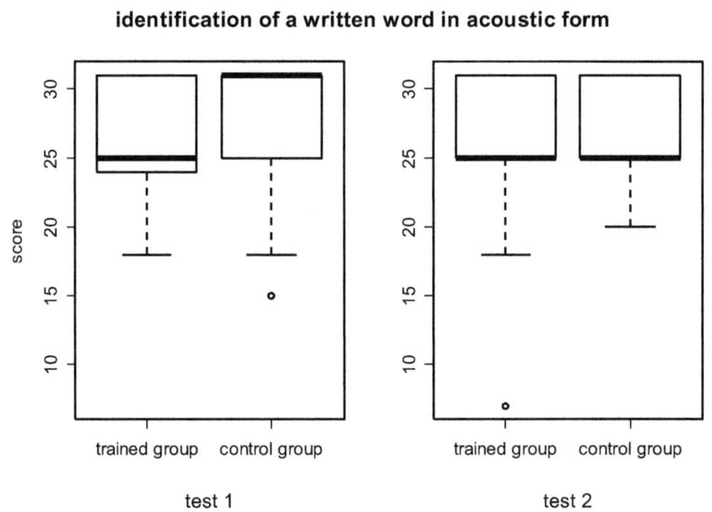

figure A.1-29: boxplots on the scores achieved in question category five in tests 1 and 2 by the two groups

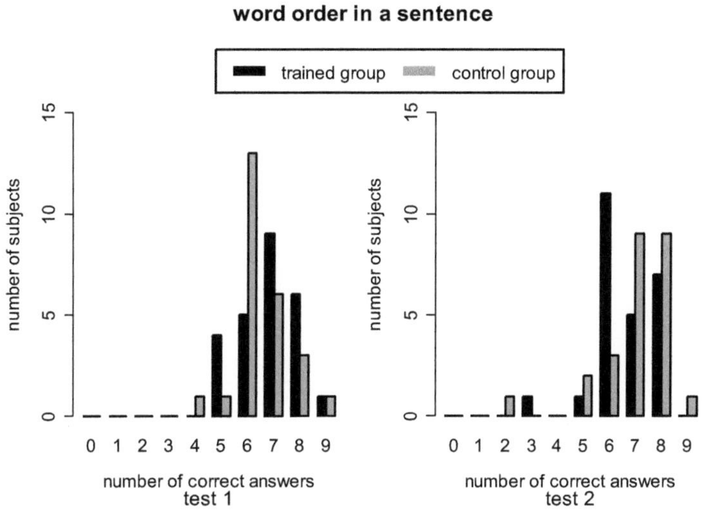

figure A.1-30: barplots on the number of category-six questions answered correctly in tests 1 and 2 by the two groups

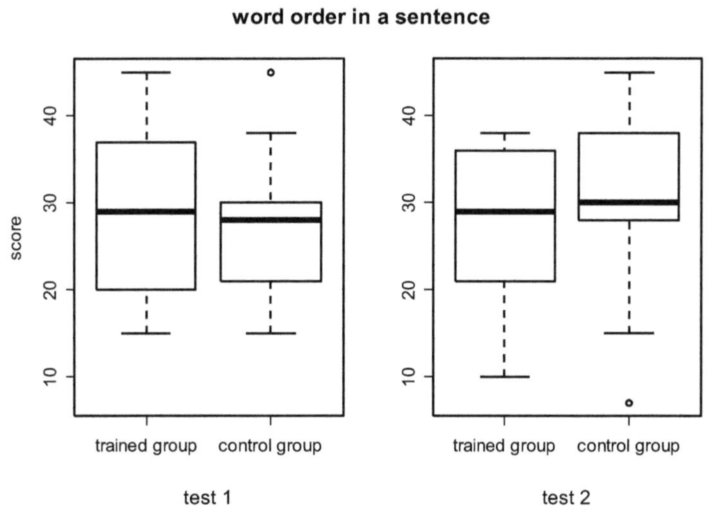

figure A.1-31: boxplots on the scores achieved in question category six in tests 1 and 2 by the two groups

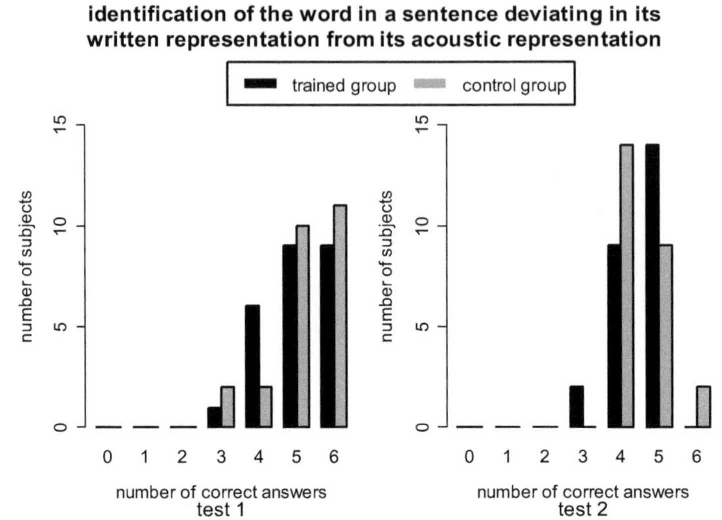

figure A.1-32: barplots on the number of category-seven questions answered correctly in tests 1 and 2 by the two groups

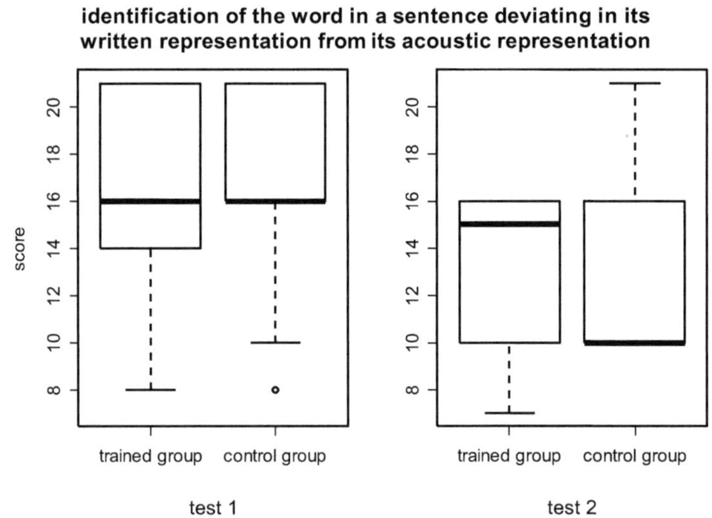

figure A.1-33: boxplots on the scores achieved in question category seven in tests 1 and 2 by the two groups

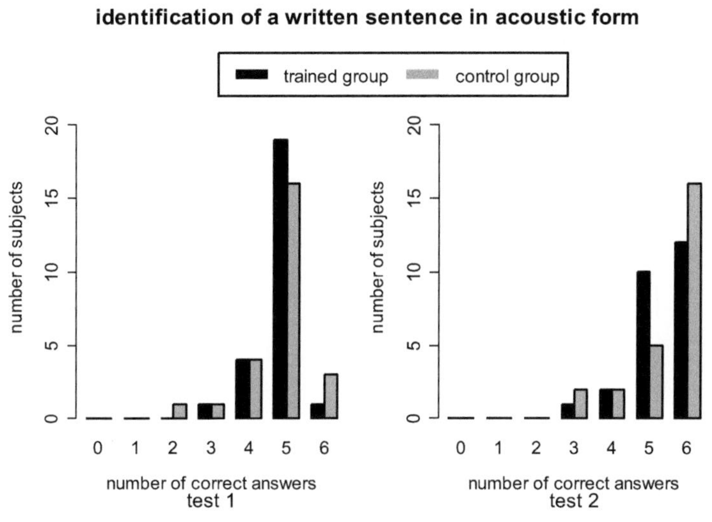

figure A.1-34: barplots on the number of category-eight questions answered correctly in tests 1 and 2 by the two groups

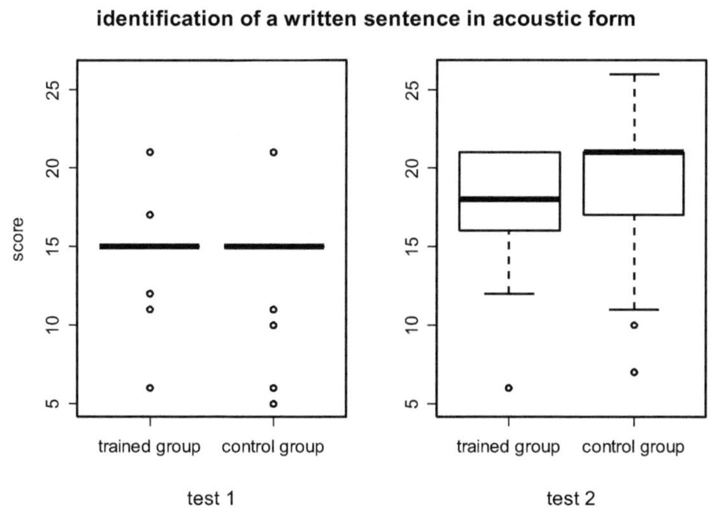

figure A.1-35: boxplots on the scores achieved in question category eight in tests 1 and 2 by the two groups

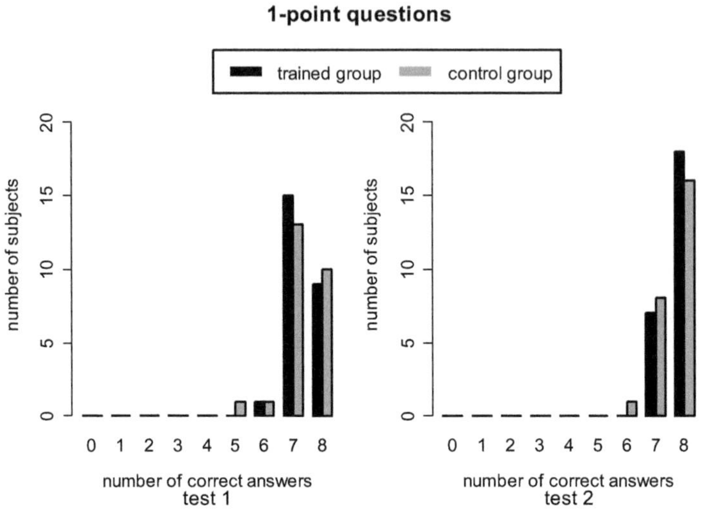

figure A.1-36: barplots on the number of difficulty-grade-one questions answered correctly in tests 1 and 2 by the two groups

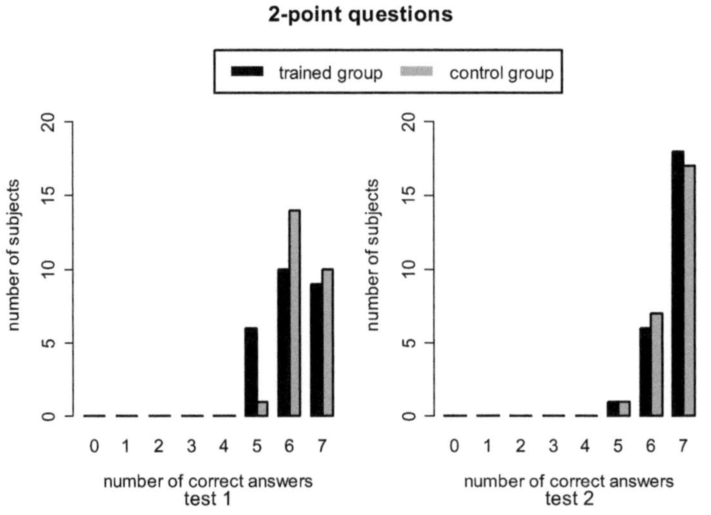

figure A.1-37: barplots on the number of difficulty-grade-two questions answered correctly in tests 1 and 2 by the two groups

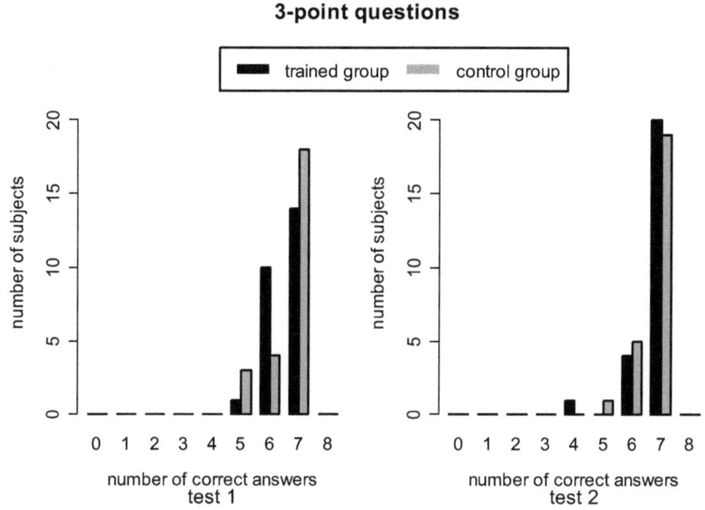

figure A.1-38: barplots on the number of difficulty-grade-three questions answered correctly in tests 1 and 2 by the two groups

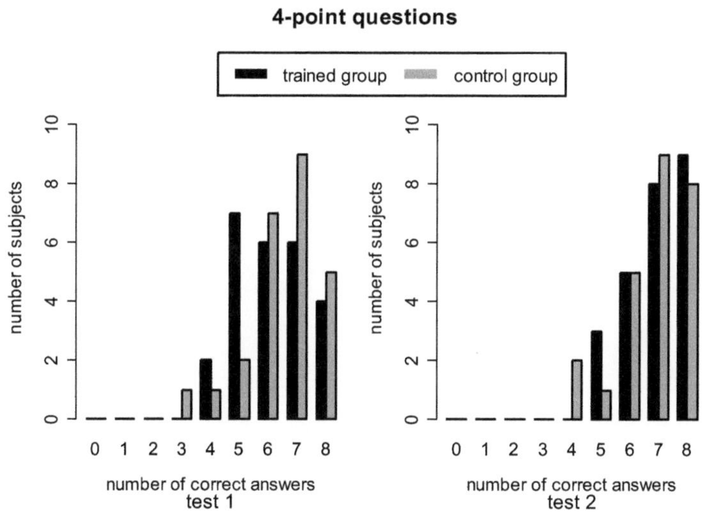

figure A.1-39: barplots on the number of difficulty-grade-four questions answered correctly in tests 1 and 2 by the two groups

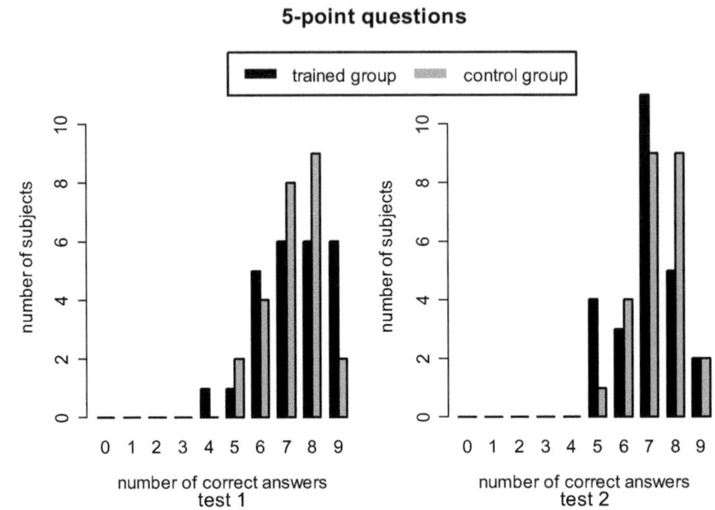

figure A.1-40: barplots on the number of difficulty-grade-five questions answered correctly in tests 1 and 2 by the two groups

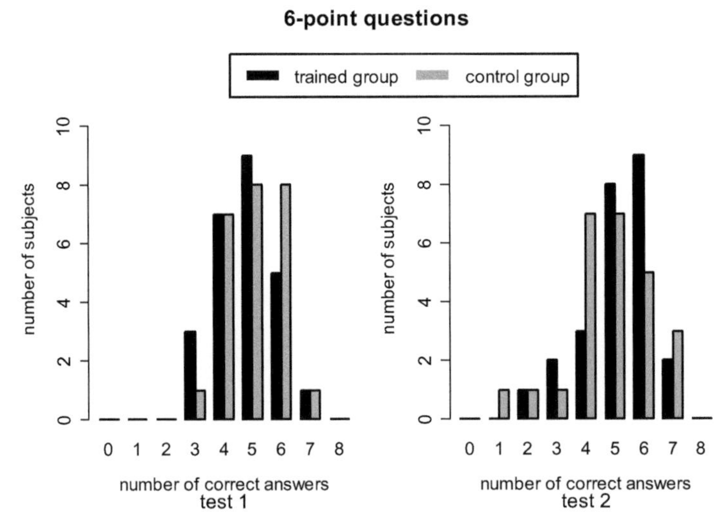

figure A.1-41: barplots on the number of difficulty-grade-six questions answered correctly in tests 1 and 2 by the two groups

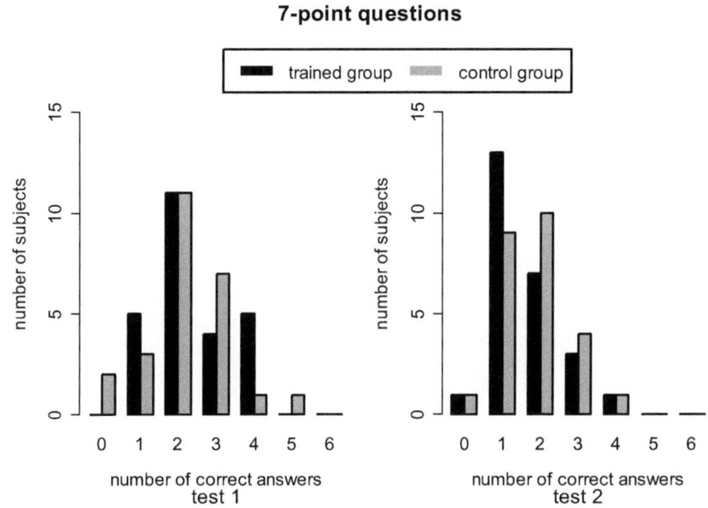

figure A.1-42: barplots on the number of difficulty-grade-seven questions answered correctly in tests 1 and 2 by the two groups

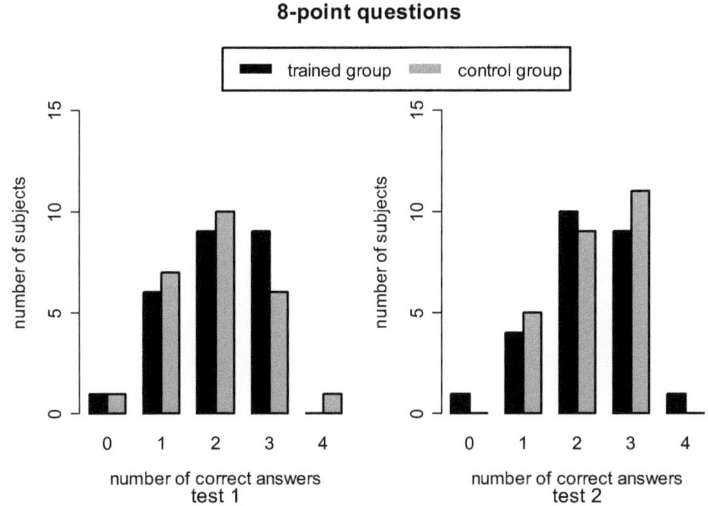

figure A.1-43: barplots on the number of difficulty-grade-eight questions answered correctly in tests 1 and 2 by the two groups

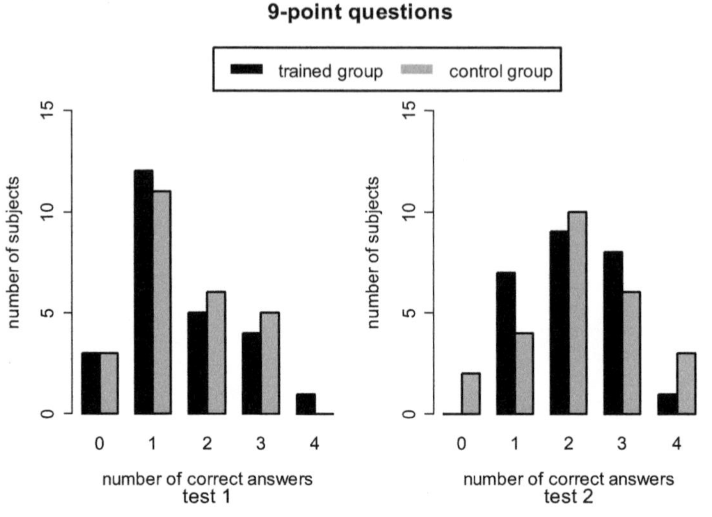

figure A.1-44: barplots on the number of difficulty-grade-nine questions answered correctly in tests 1 and 2 by the two groups

Appendix A.2 Barplots on the Answer Frequencies in the Subjects' Self-Evaluation

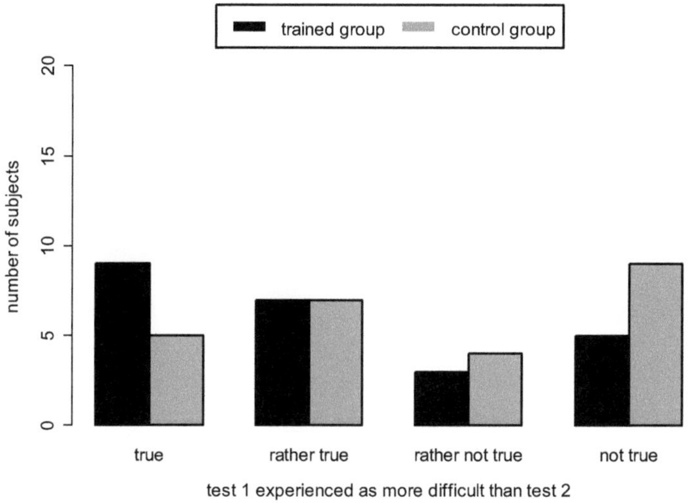

figure A.2-45: answer frequencies for the statement of test 1 experienced as more difficult than test 2

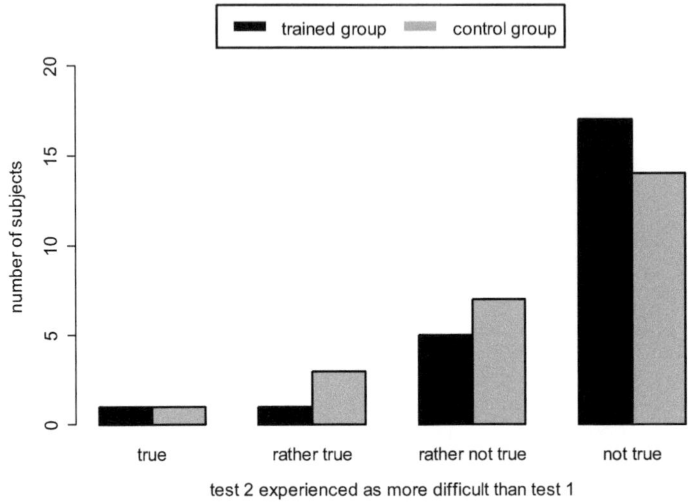

figure A.2-46: answer frequencies for the statement of test 2 experienced as more difficult than test 1

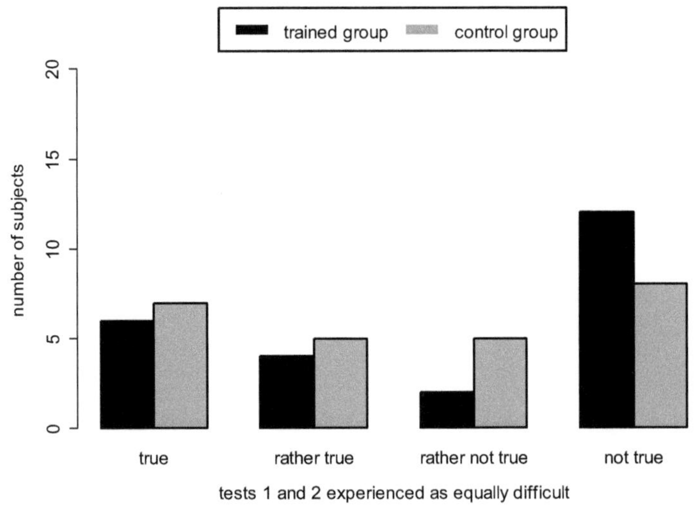

figure A.2-47: answer frequencies for the statement of test 1 and 2 experienced as equally difficult

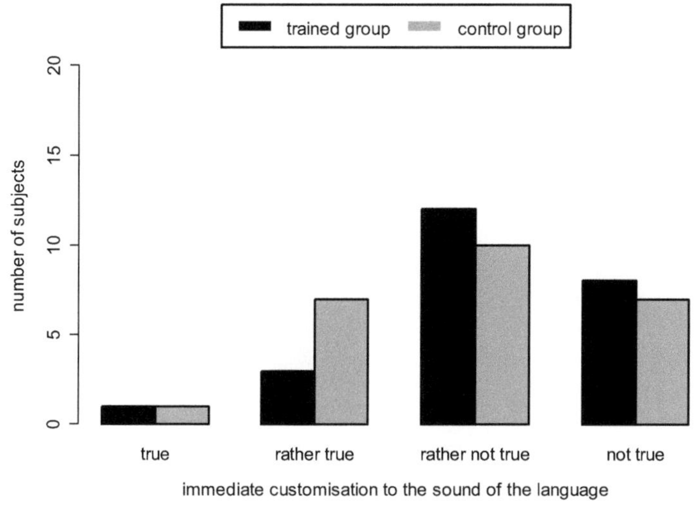

figure A.2-48: answer frequencies for the statement of the subjects' immediate accustomisation to the sound of the language

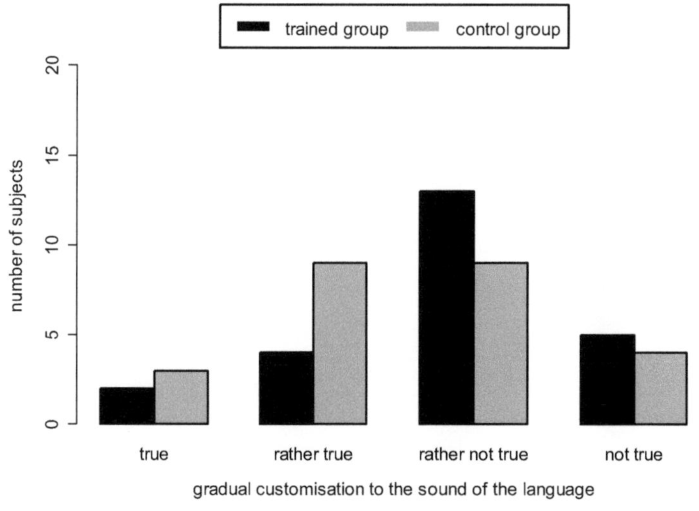

figure A.2-49: answer frequencies for the statement of the subjects' gradual accustomisation to the sound of the language

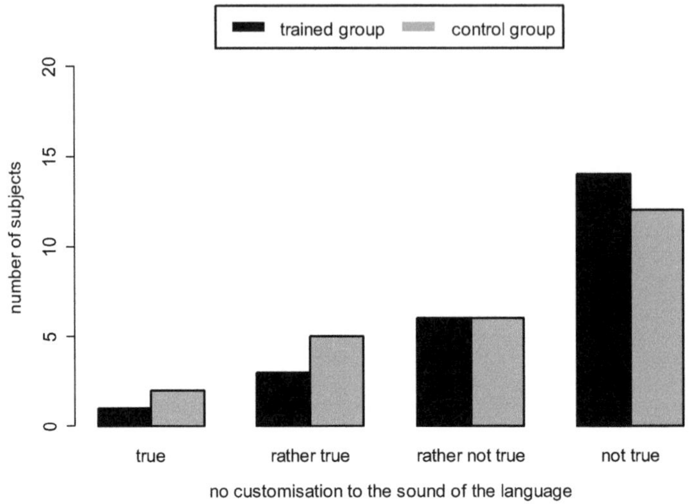

figure A.2-50: answer frequencies for the statement of the subjects' inability to adapt to the sound of the language

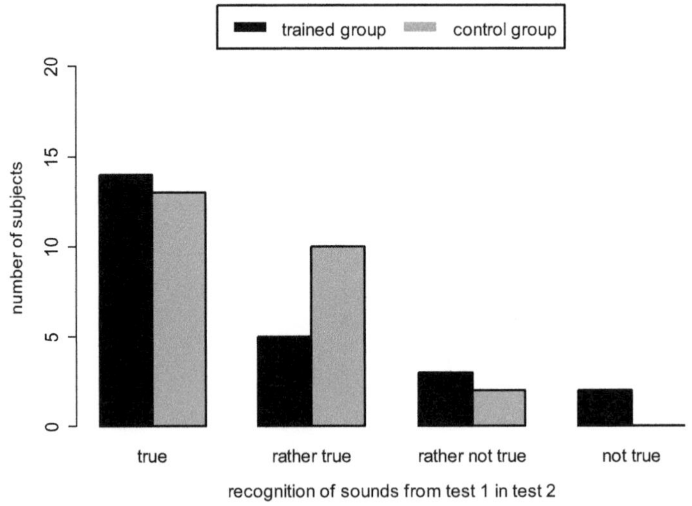

figure A.1-51: answer frequencies for the statement of the subjects recognising sounds from test 1 in test 2

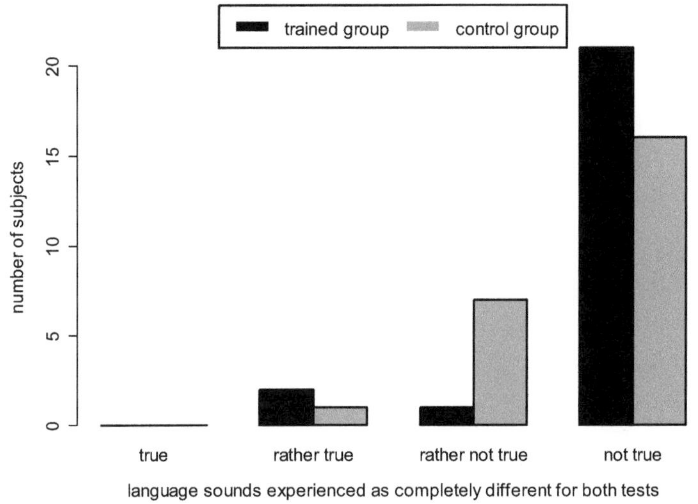

figure A.2-52: answer frequencies for the statement of language sounds experienced as completely different for both tests

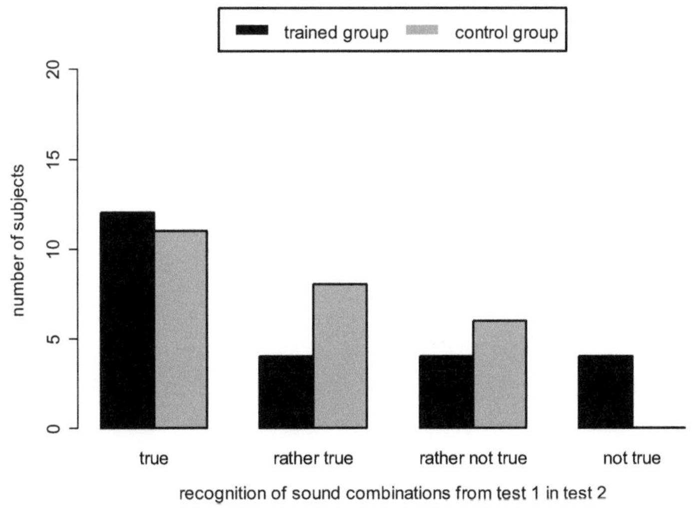

figure A.2-53: answer frequencies for the statement of the subjects recognising sound combinations from test 1 in test 2

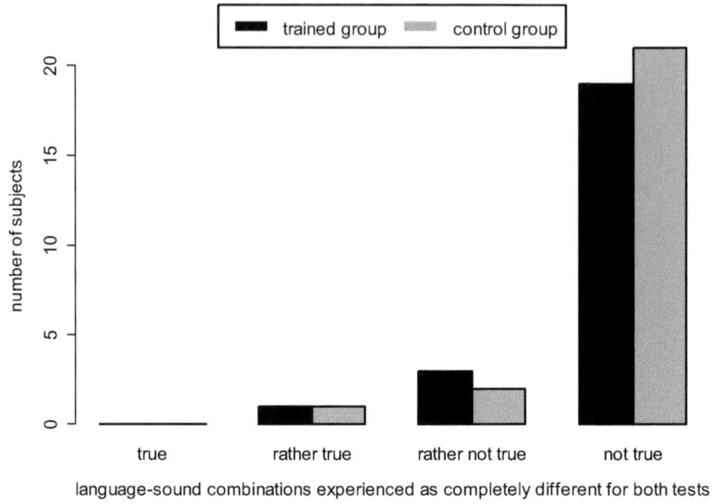

figure A.2-54: answer frequencies for the statement of language-sound combinations experienced as completely different for both tests

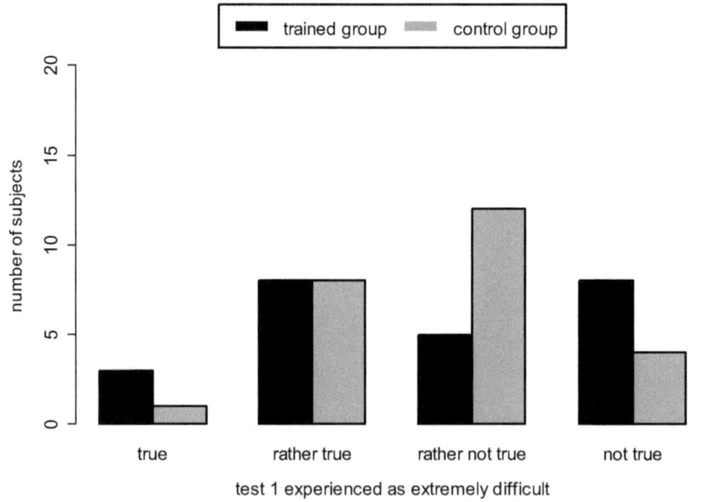

figure A.1-55: answer frequencies for the statement of test 1 experienced as extremely difficult

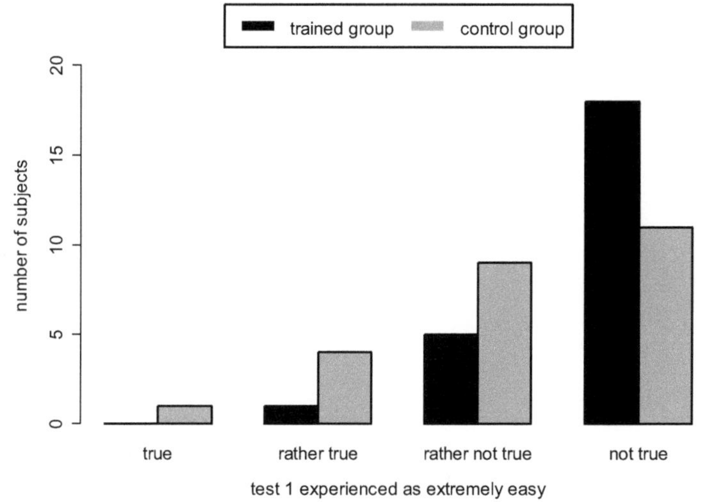

figure A.2-56: answer frequencies for the statement of test 1 experienced as extremely easy

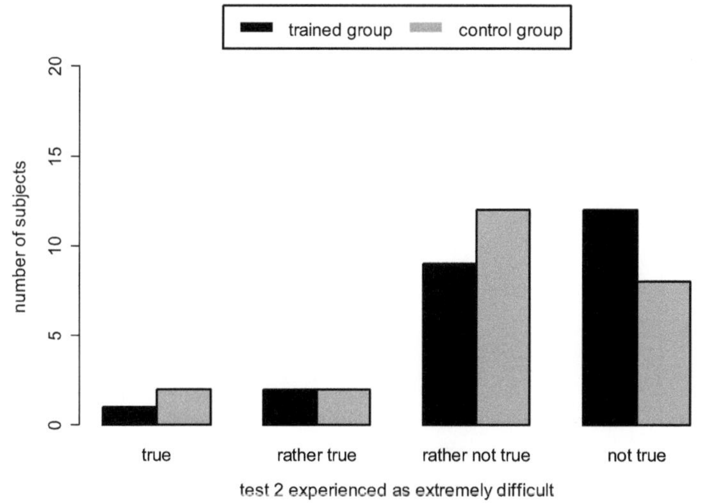

figure A.2-57: answer frequencies for the statement of test 2 experienced as extremely difficult

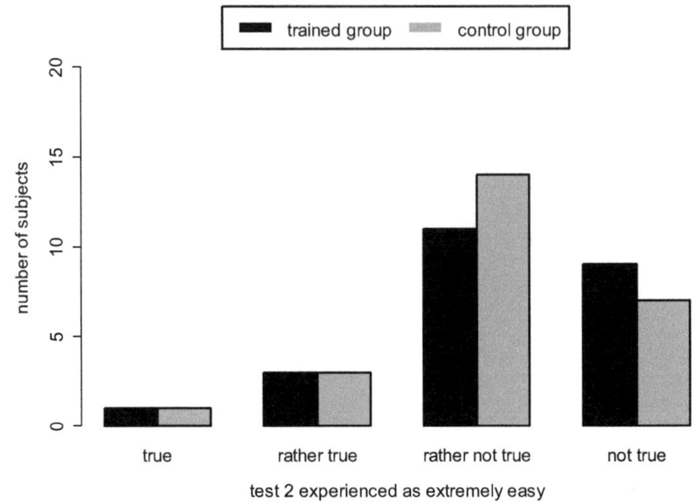

figure A.2-58: answer frequencies for the statement of test 2 experienced as extremely easy

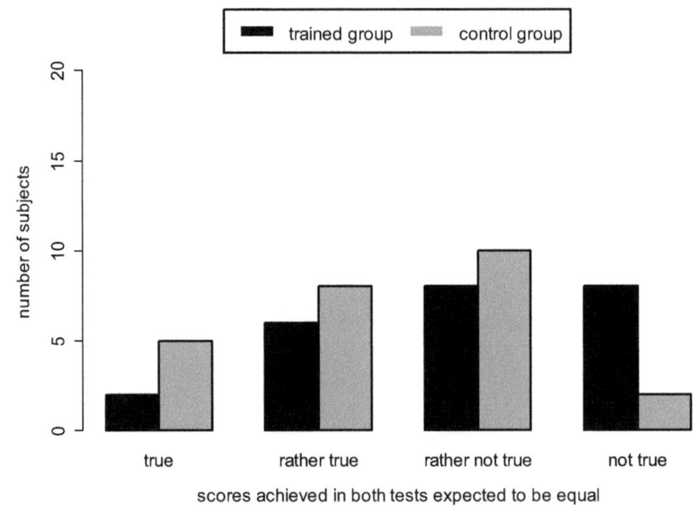

figure A.2-59: answer frequencies for the statement of the scores achieved in both tests expected to be equal

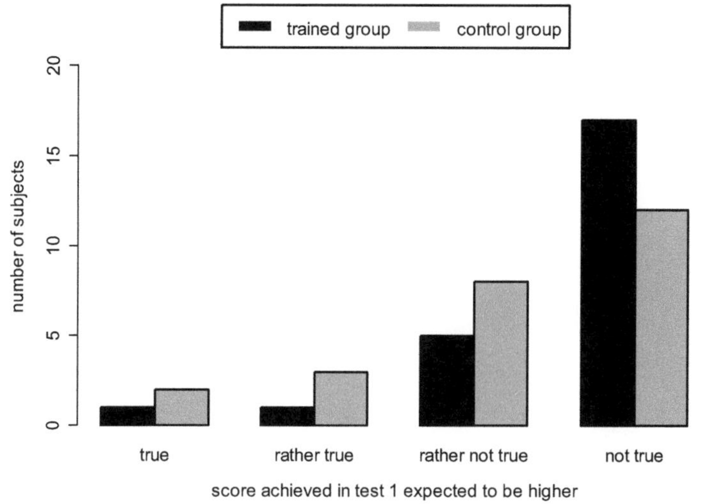

figure A.2-60: answer frequencies for the statement of the score achieved in test 1 expected to be higher

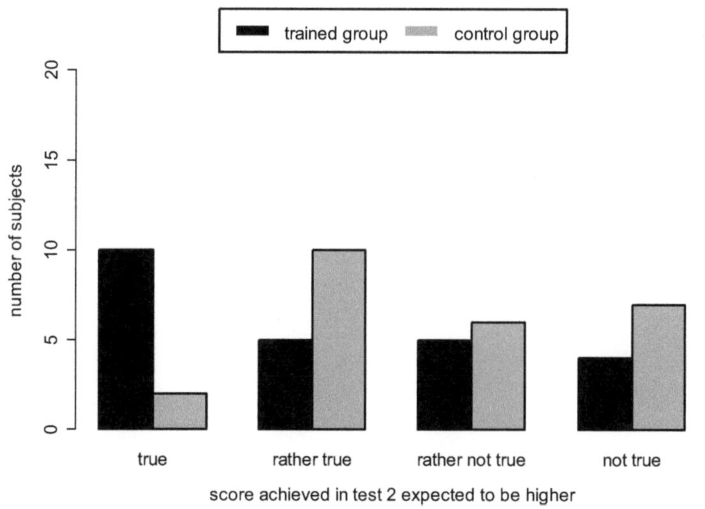

figure A.2-61: answer frequencies for the statement of the score achieved in test 2 expected to be higher

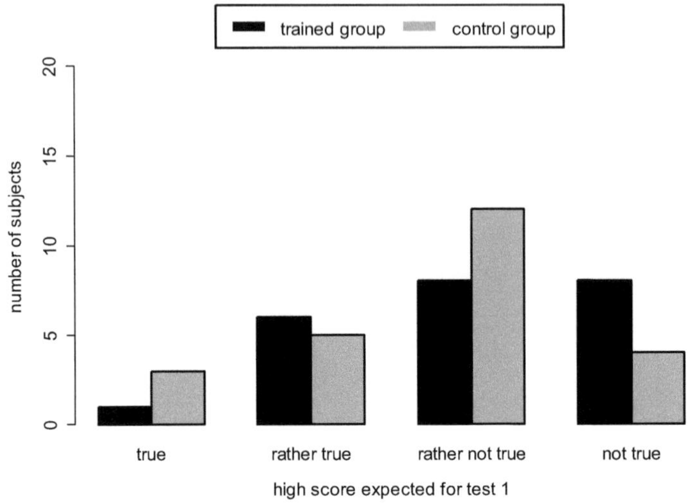

figure A.2-62: answer frequencies for the statement of a high score expected for test 1

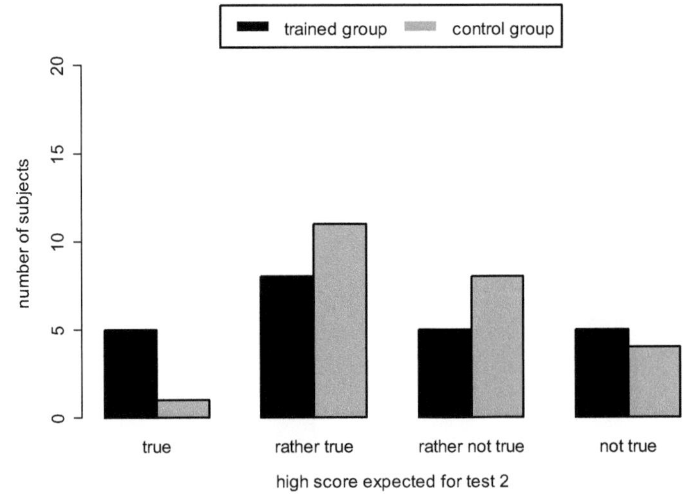

figure A.2-63: answer frequencies for the statement of a high score expected for test 2

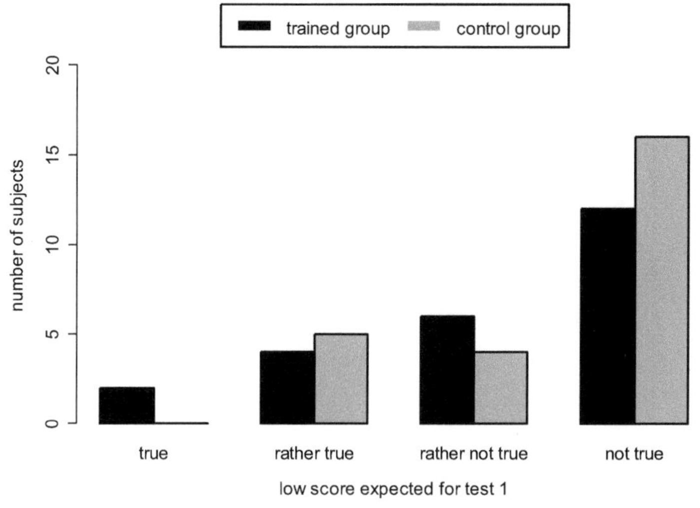

figure A.2-64: answer frequencies for the statement of a low score expected for test 1

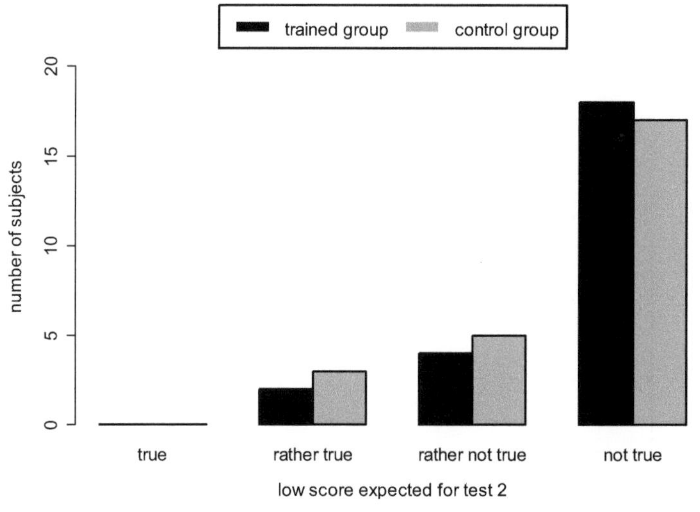

figure A.2-65: answer frequencies for the statement of a low score expected for test 2

Appendix A.3 Graphs on the Correlation between the Subjects' Self-Evaluation and Test Performance

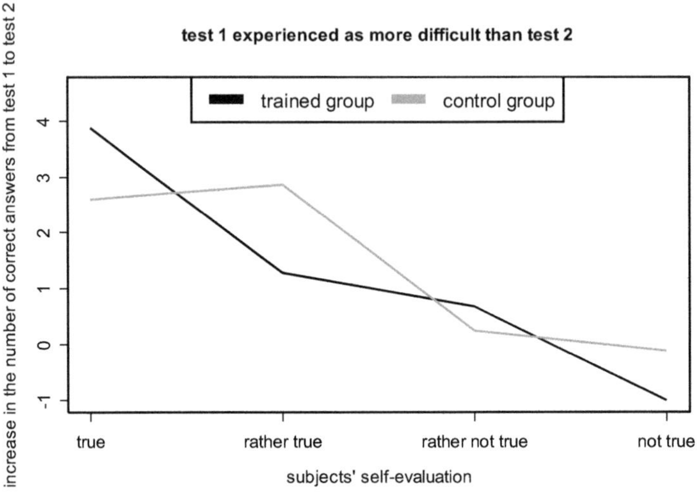

figure A.3-66: responses to the statement of test 1 experienced as more difficult than test 2 juxtaposed with the increase in the number of correct answers

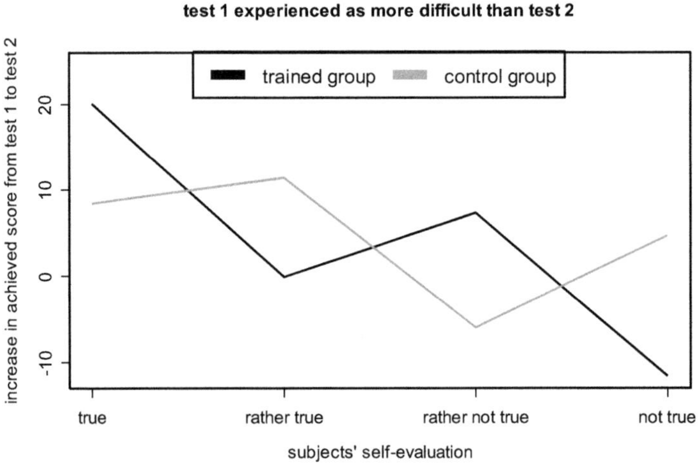

figure A.3-67: responses to the statement of test 1 experienced as more difficult than test 2 juxtaposed with the increase in the achieved score

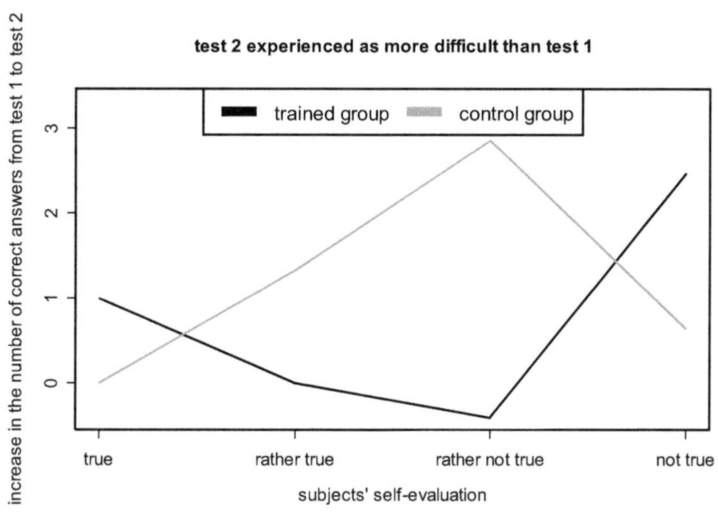

figure A.3-68: responses to the statement of test 2 experienced as more difficult than test 1 juxtaposed with the increase in the number of correct answers

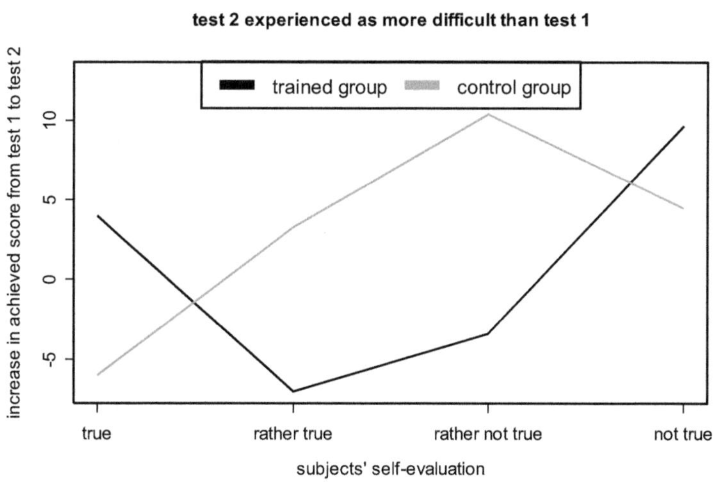

figure A.3-69: responses to the statement of test 2 experienced as more difficult than test 1 juxtaposed with the increase in the achieved score

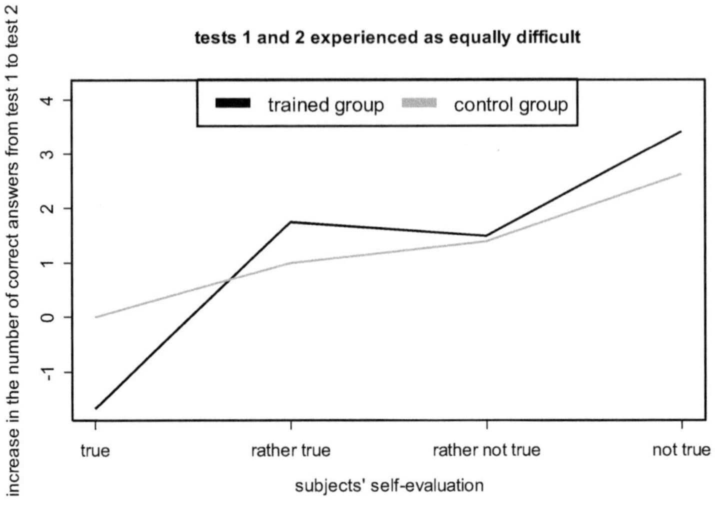

figure A.3-70: responses to the statement of test 1 and 2 experienced as equally difficult juxtaposed with the increase in the number of correct answers

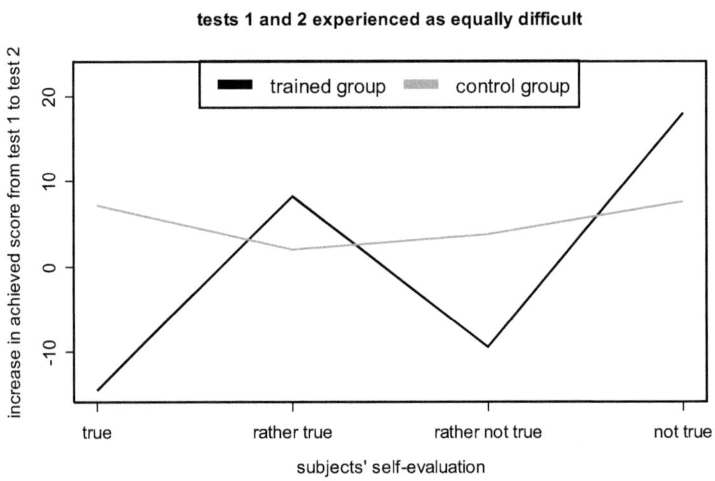

figure A.3-71: responses to the statement of test 1 and 2 experienced as equally difficult juxtaposed with the increase in the achieved score

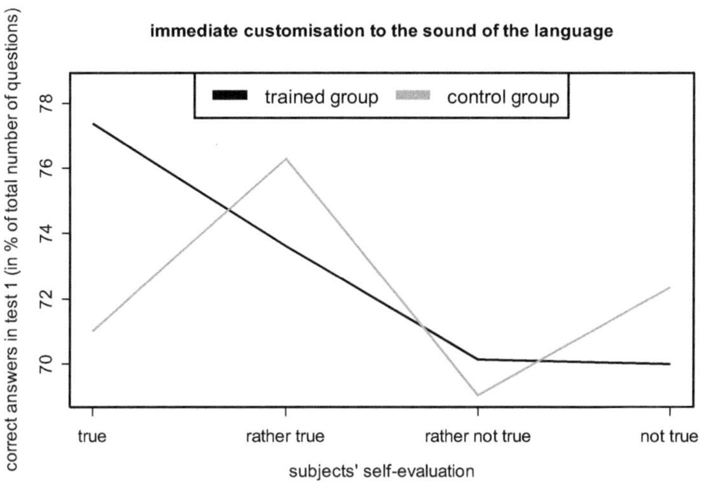

figure A.3-72: responses to the statement of the subjects' immediate accustomisation to the sound of the language juxtaposed with the percentage of questions answered correctly in test 1

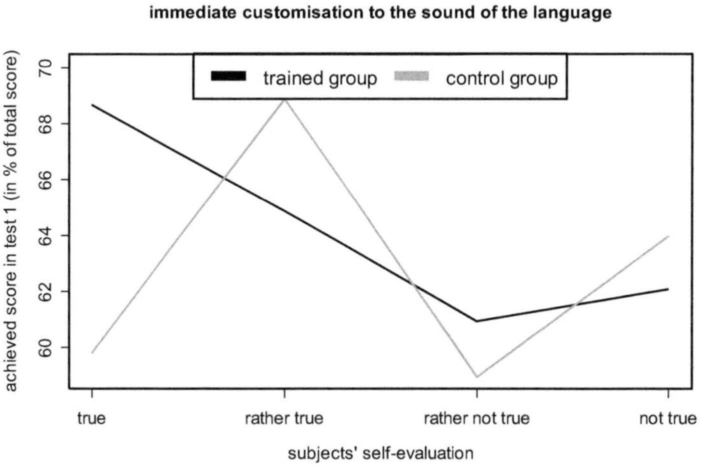

figure A.3-73: responses to the statement of the subjects' immediate accustomisation to the sound of the language juxtaposed with the percentage of the maximum score achieved in test 1

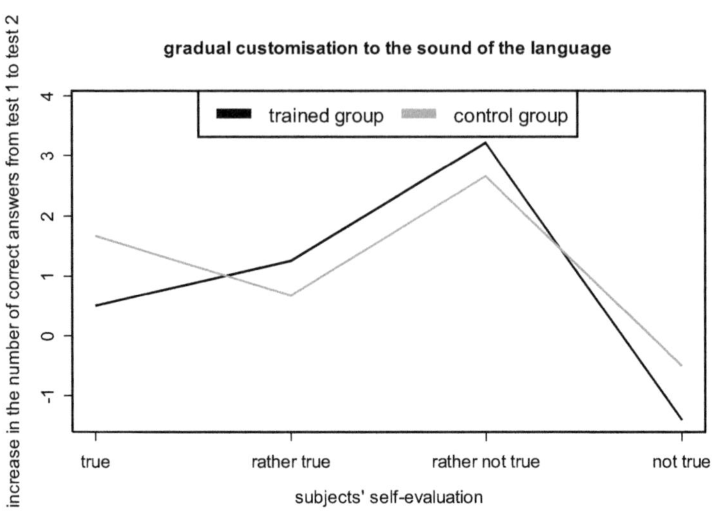

figure A.3-74: responses to the statement of the subjects' gradual accustomisation to the sound of the language juxtaposed with the increase in the number of correct answers

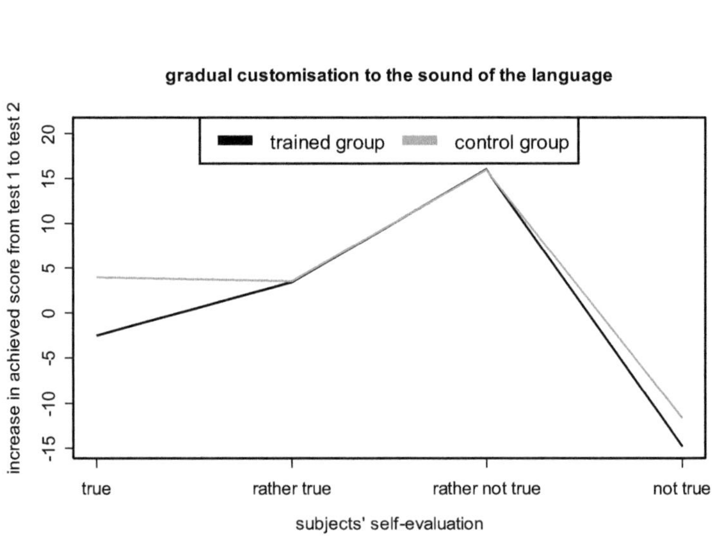

figure A.3-75: responses to the statement of the subjects' gradual accustomisation to the sound of the language juxtaposed with the increase in the achieved score

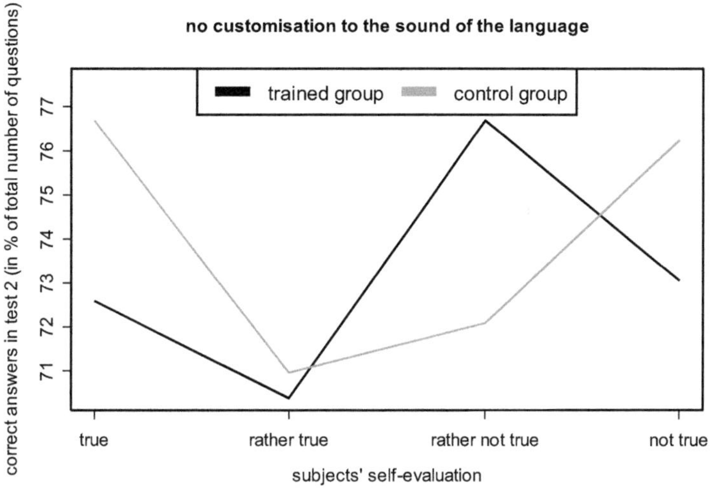

figure A.3-76: responses to the statement of the subjects' inability to adapt to the sound of the language juxtaposed with the percentage of questions answered correctly in test 2

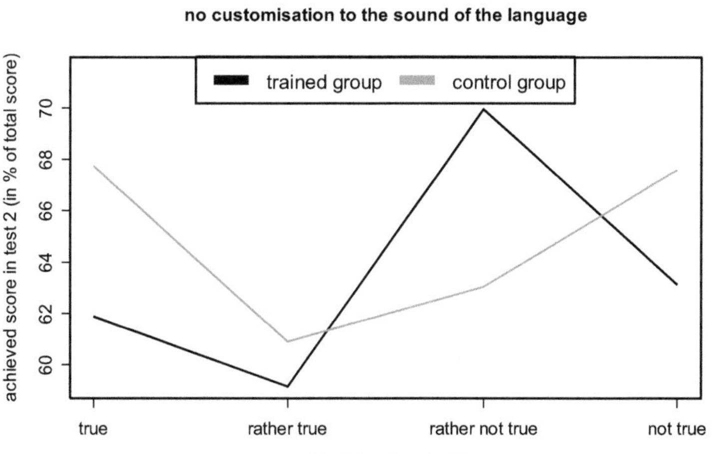

figure A.3-77: responses to the statement of the subjects' inability to adapt to the sound of the language juxtaposed with the percentage of the maximum score achieved in test 2

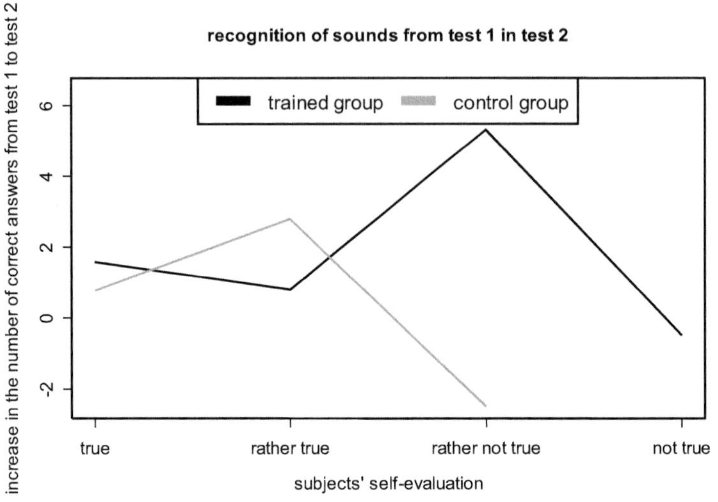

figure A.3-78: responses to the statement of the subjects recognising sounds from test 1 in test 2 juxtaposed with the increase in the number of correct answers

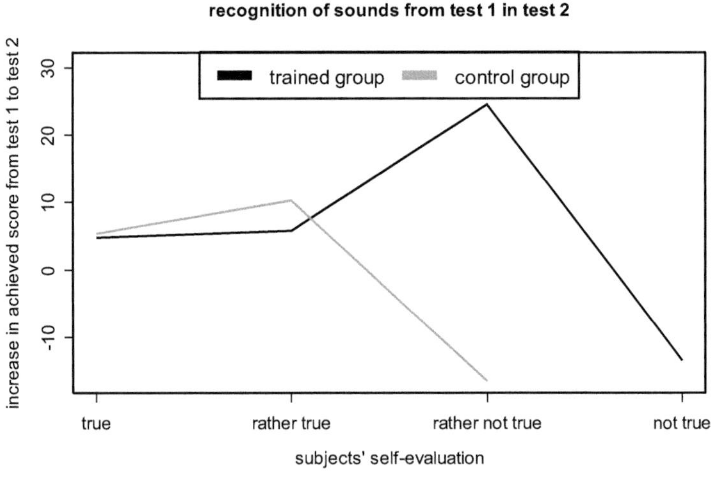

figure A.3-79: responses to the statement of the subjects recognising sounds from test 1 in test 2 juxtaposed with the increase in the achieved score

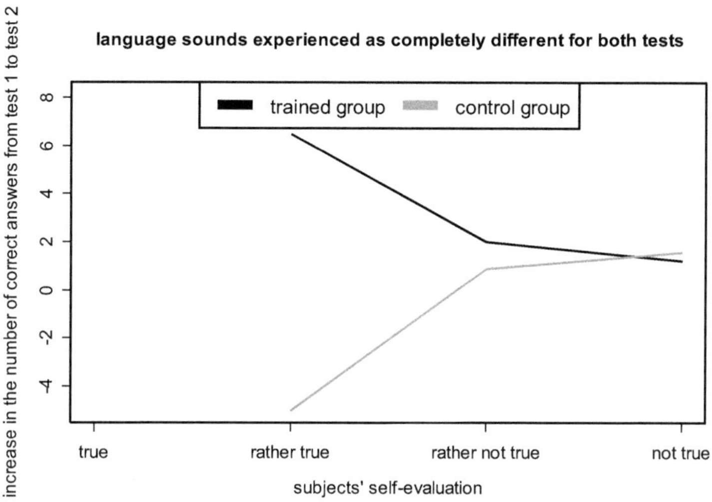

figure A.3-80: responses to the statement of the language sounds experienced as completely different for both tests juxtaposed with the increase in the number of correct answers

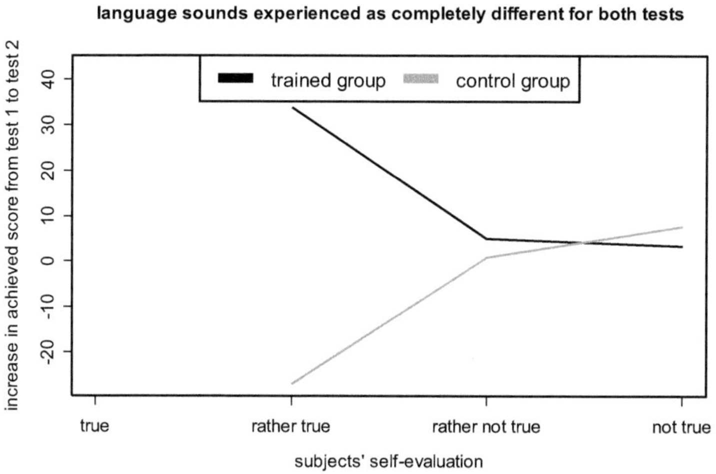

figure A.3-81: responses to the statement of the language sounds experienced as completely different for both tests juxtaposed with the increase in the achieved score

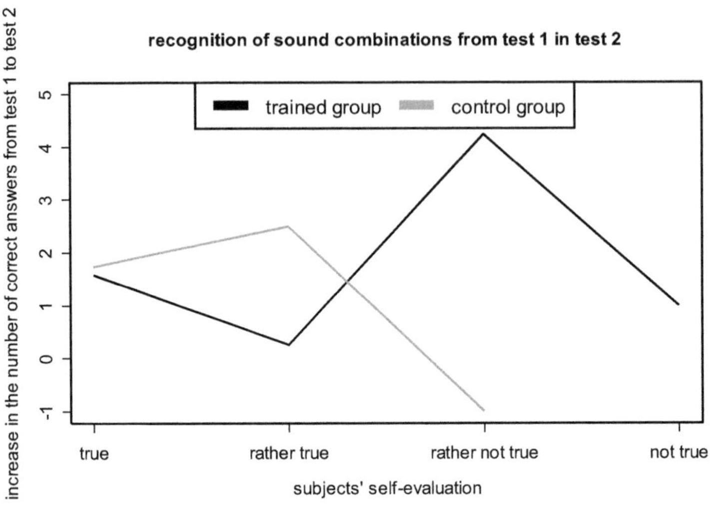

figure A.3-82: responses to the statement of the subjects recognising sound combinations from test 1 in test 2 juxtaposed with the increase in the number of correct answers

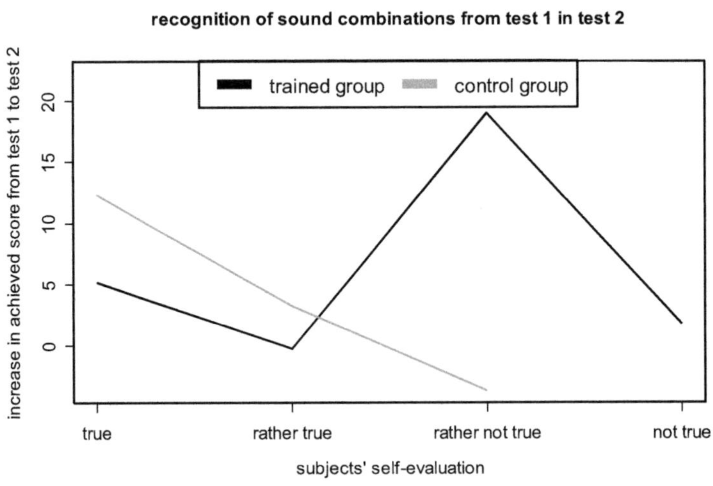

figure A.3-83: responses to the statement of the subjects recognising sound combinations from test 1 in test 2 juxtaposed with the increase in the achieved score

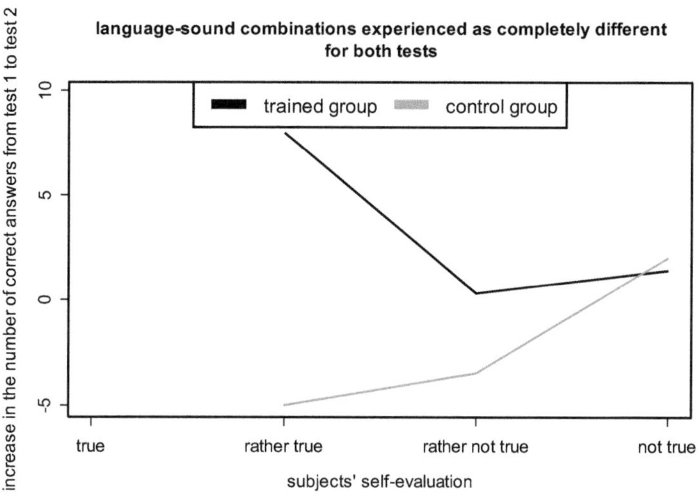

figure A.3-84: responses to the statement of the language-sound combinations experienced as completely different for both tests juxtaposed with the increase in the number of correct answers

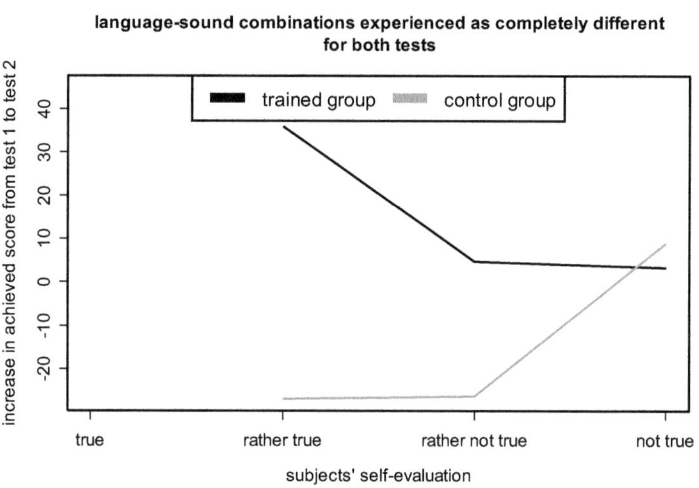

figure A.3-85: responses to the statement of the language-sound combinations experienced as completely different for both tests juxtaposed with the increase in the achieved score

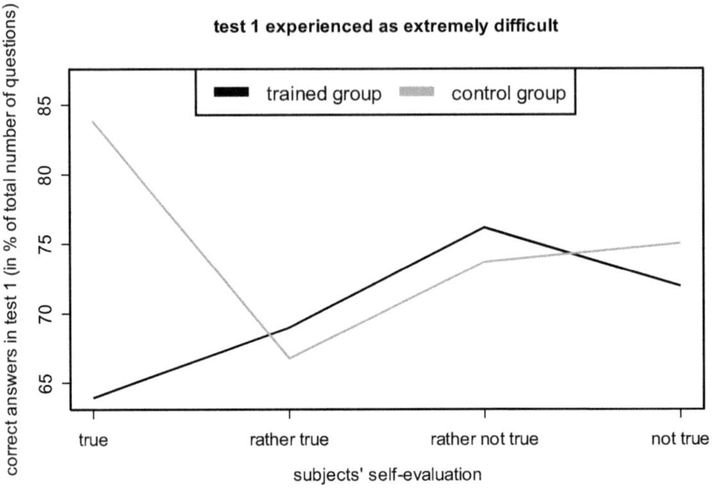

figure A.3-86: responses to the statement of test 1 experienced as extremely difficult juxtaposed with the percentage of questions answered correctly in test 1

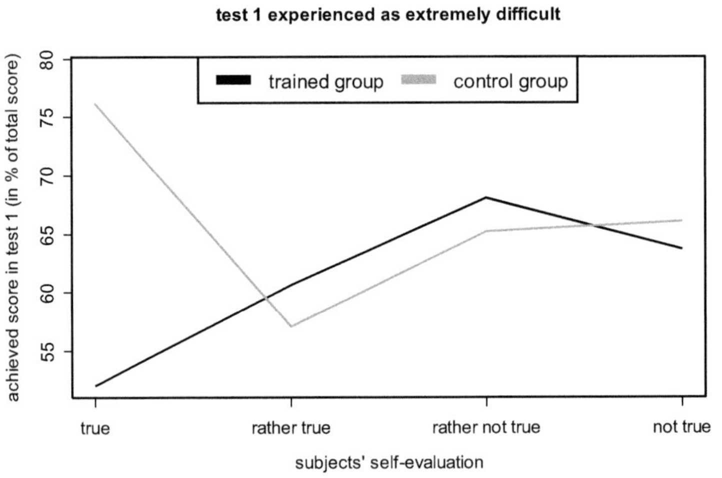

figure A.3-87: responses to the statement of test 1 experienced as extremely difficult juxtaposed with the percentage of the maximum score achieved in test 1

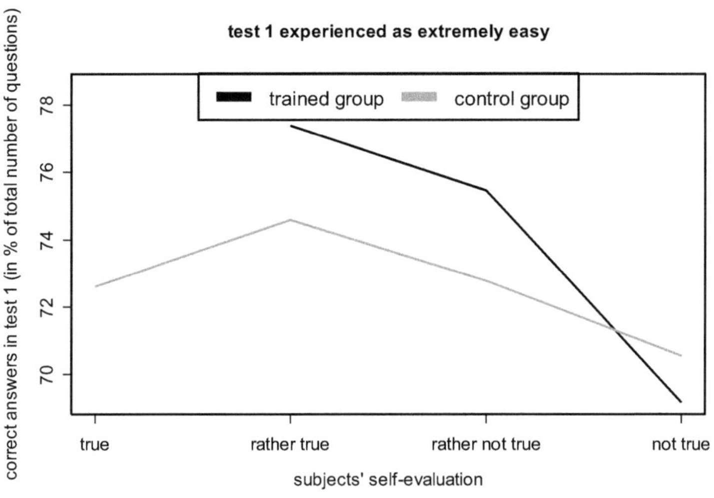

figure A.3-88: responses to the statement of test 1 experienced as extremely easy juxtaposed with the percentage of questions answered correctly in test 1

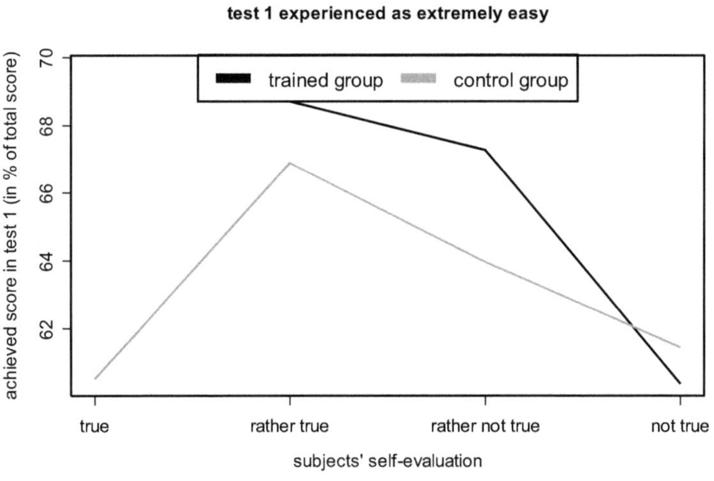

figure A.3-89: responses to the statement of test 1 experienced as extremely easy juxtaposed with the percentage of the maximum score achieved in test 1

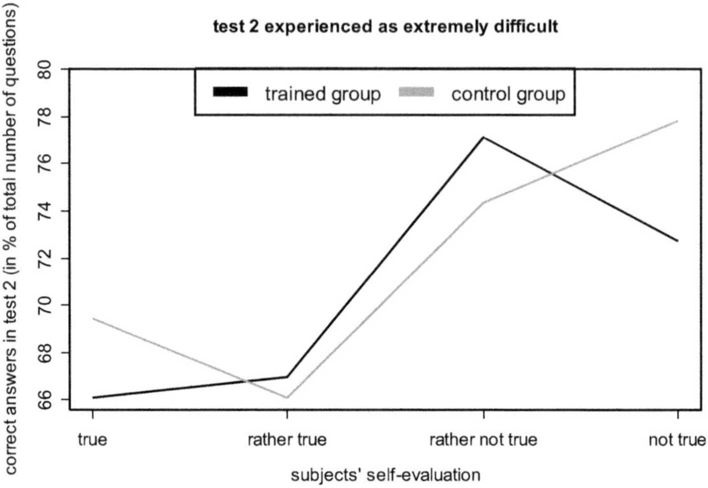

figure A.3-90: responses to the statement of test 2 experienced as extremely difficult juxtaposed with the percentage of questions answered correctly in test 2

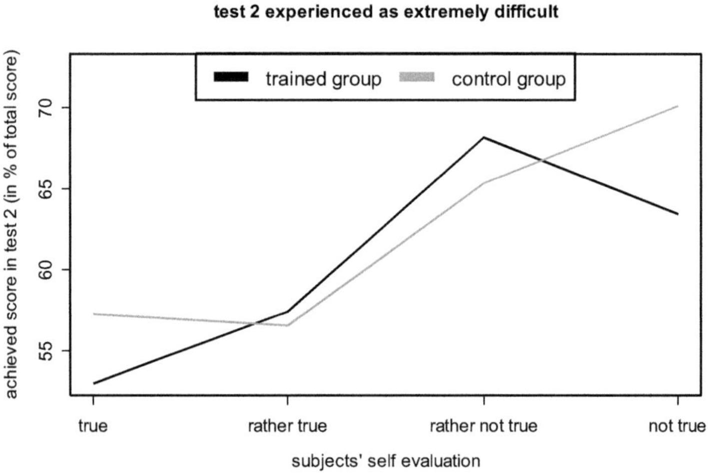

figure A.3-91: responses to the statement of test 2 experienced as extremely difficult juxtaposed with the percentage of the maximum score achieved in test 2

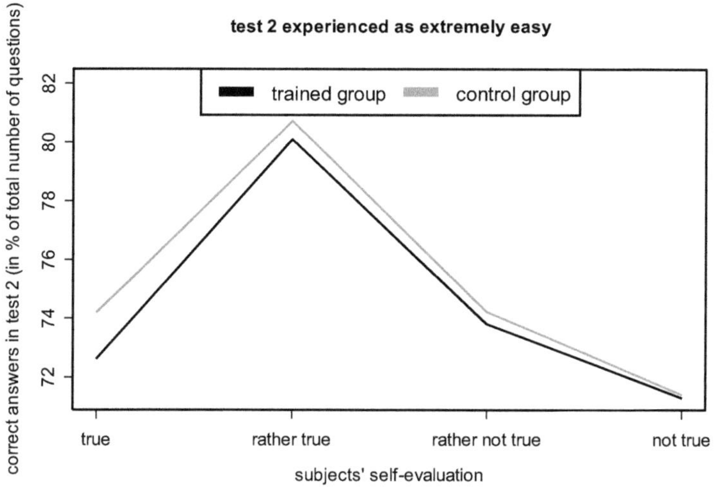

figure A.3-92: responses to the statement of test 2 experienced as extremely easy juxtaposed with the percentage of questions answered correctly in test 2

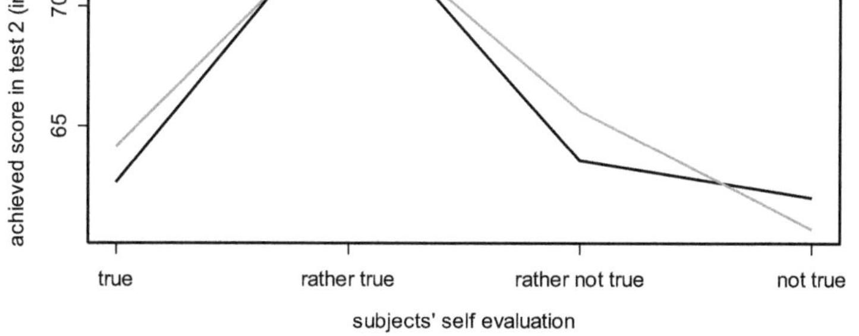

figure A.3-93: responses to the statement of test 2 experienced as extremely easy juxtaposed with the percentage of the maximum score achieved in test 2

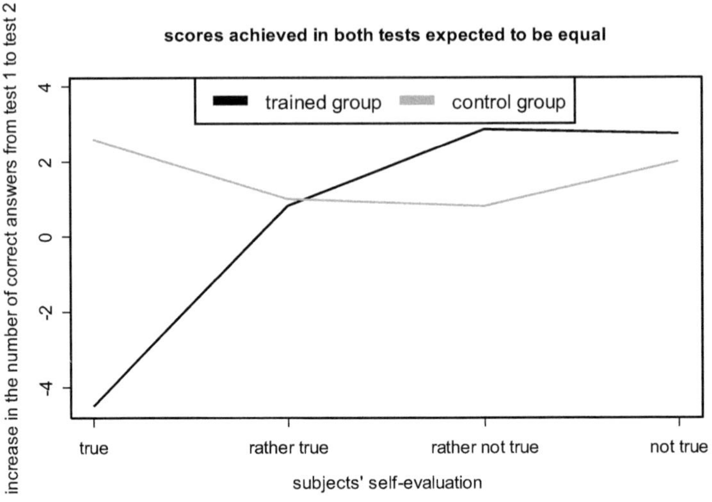

figure A.3-94: responses to the statement of the scores achieved in both tests expected to be equal juxtaposed with the increase in the number of correct answers

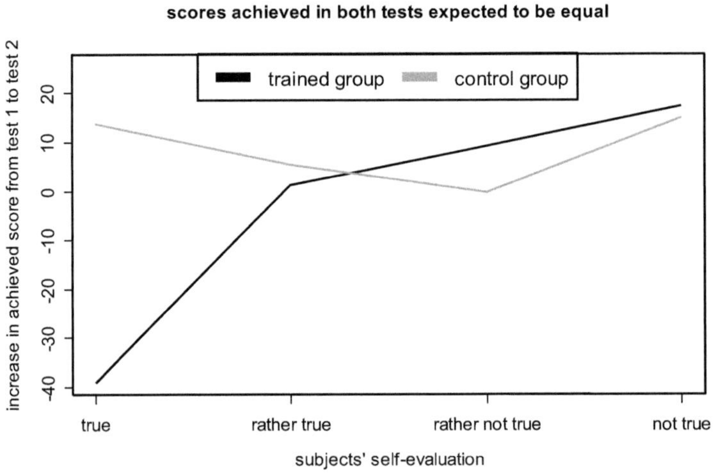

figure A.3-95: responses to the statement of the scores achieved in both tests expected to be equal juxtaposed with the increase in the achieved score

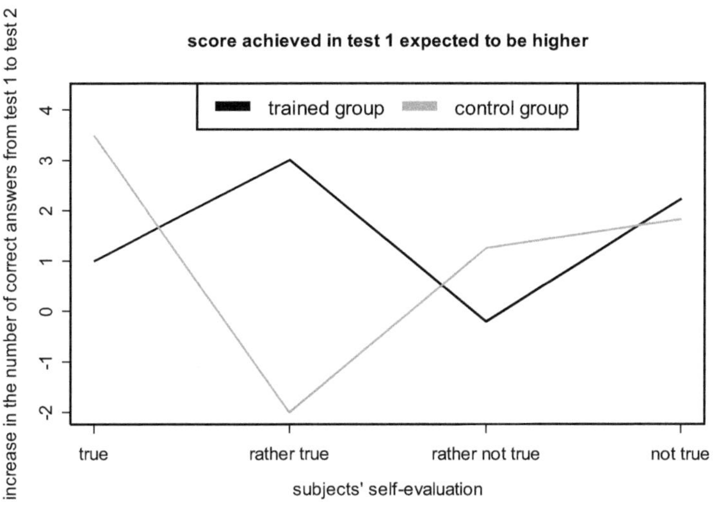

figure A.3-96: responses to the statement of the score achieved in test 1 expected to be higher juxtaposed with the increase in the number of correct answers

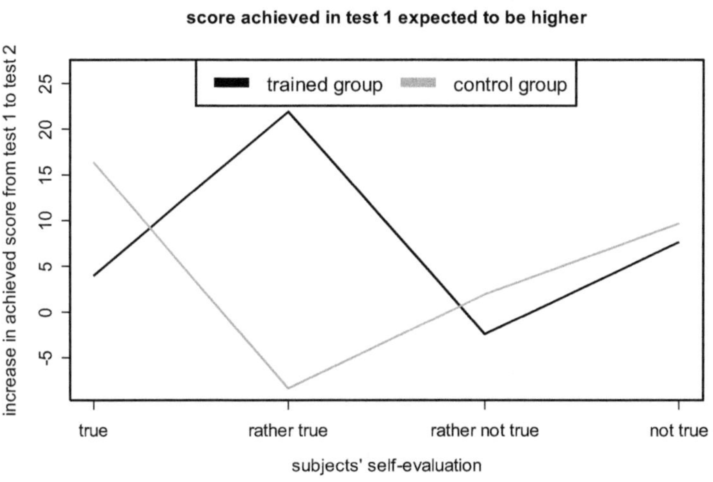

figure A.3-97: responses to the statement of the score achieved in test 1 expected to be higher juxtaposed with the increase in the achieved score

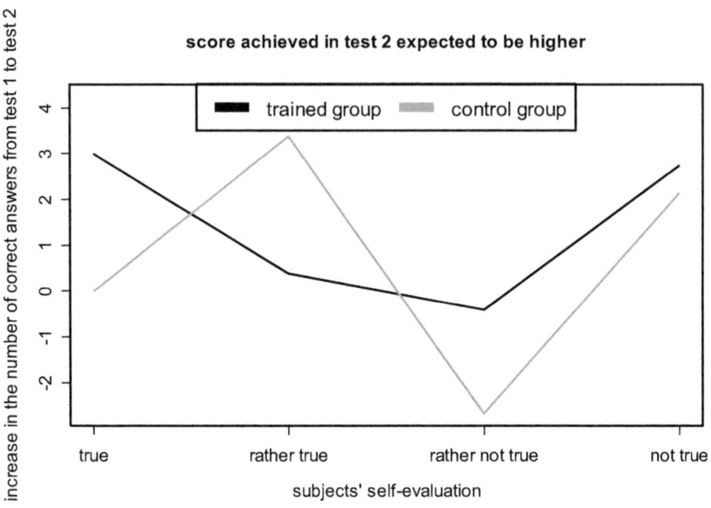

figure A.3-98: responses to the statement of the score achieved in test 2 expected to be higher juxtaposed with the increase in the number of correct answers

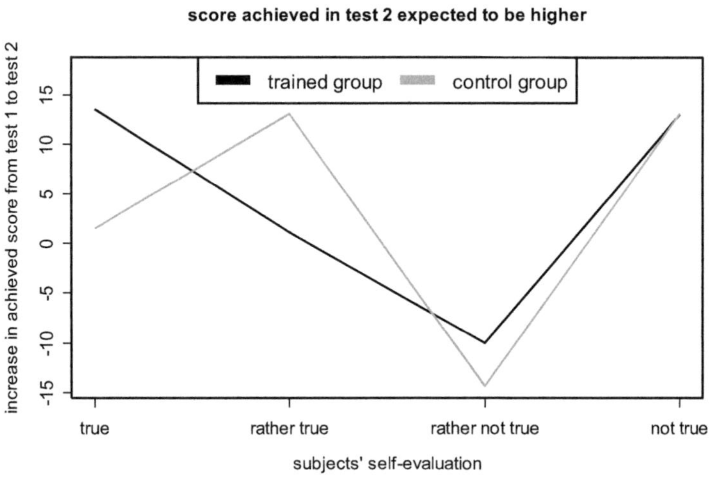

figure A.3-99: responses to the statement of the score achieved in test 2 expected to be higher juxtaposed with the increase in the achieved score

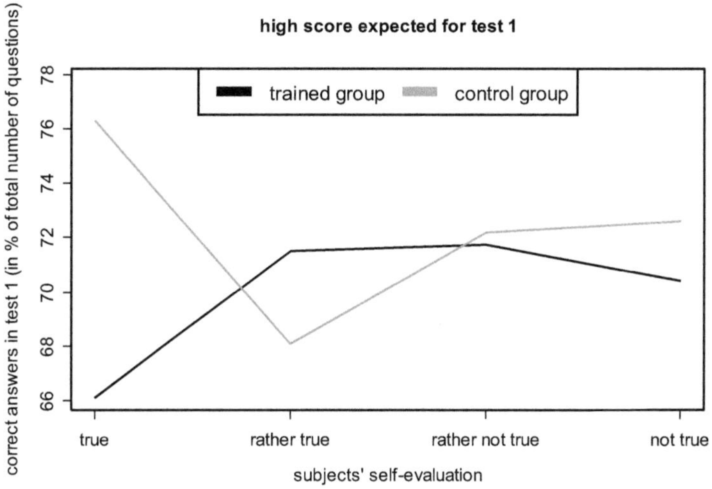

figure A.3-100: responses to the statement of a high score expected for test 1 juxtaposed with the percentage of questions answered correctly in test 1

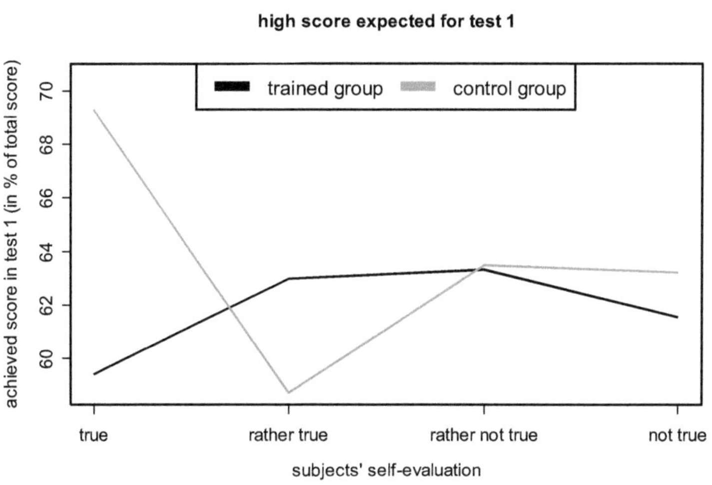

figure A.3-101: responses to the statement of a high score expected for test 1 juxtaposed with the percentage of the maximum score achieved in test 1

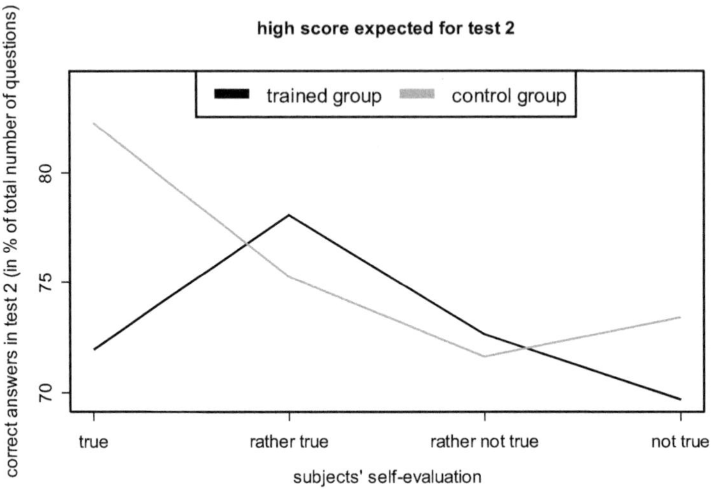

figure A.3-102: responses to the statement of a high score expected for test 2 juxtaposed with the percentage of questions answered correctly in test 2

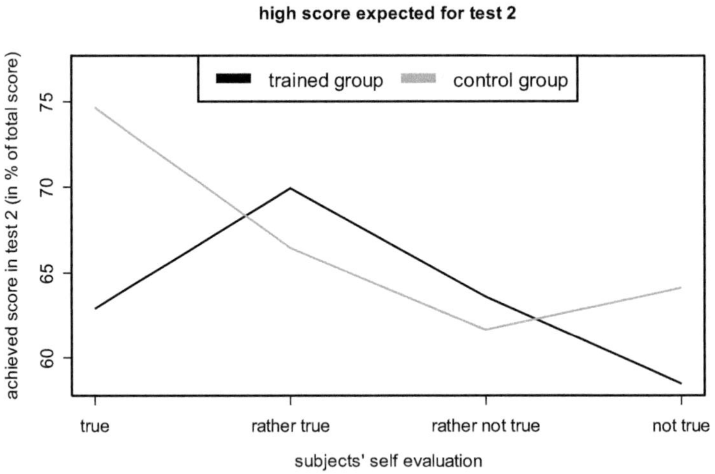

figure A.3-103: responses to the statement of a high score expected for test 2 juxtaposed with the percentage of the maximum score achieved in test 2

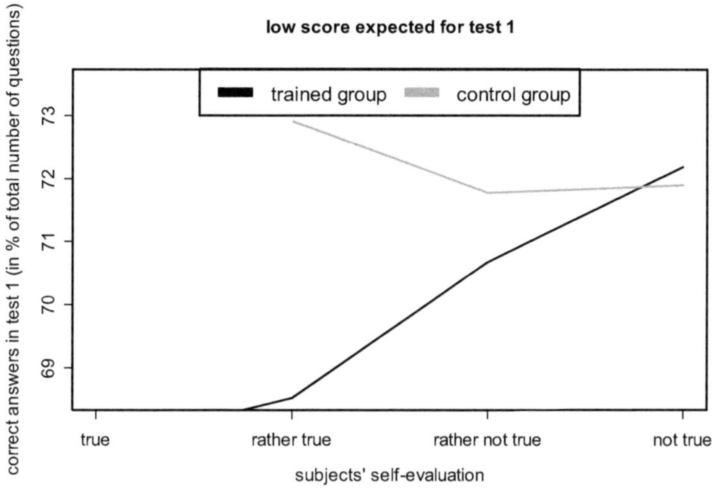

figure A.3-104: responses to the statement of a low score expected for test 1 juxtaposed with the percentage of questions answered correctly in test 1

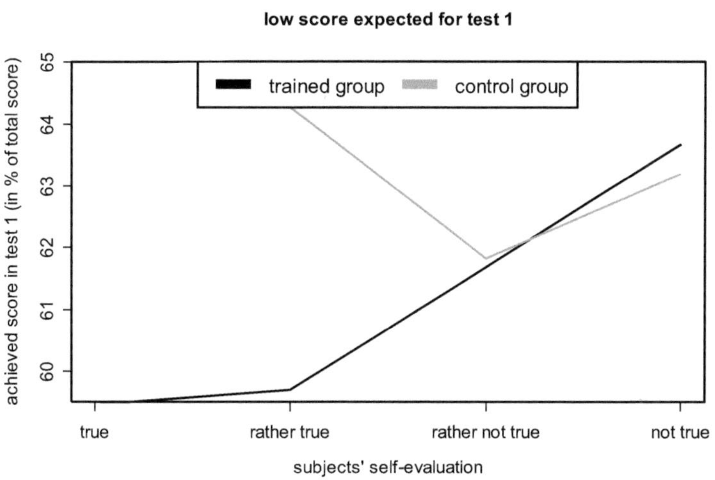

figure A.3-105: responses to the statement of a low score expected for test 1 juxtaposed with the percentage of the maximum score achieved in test 1

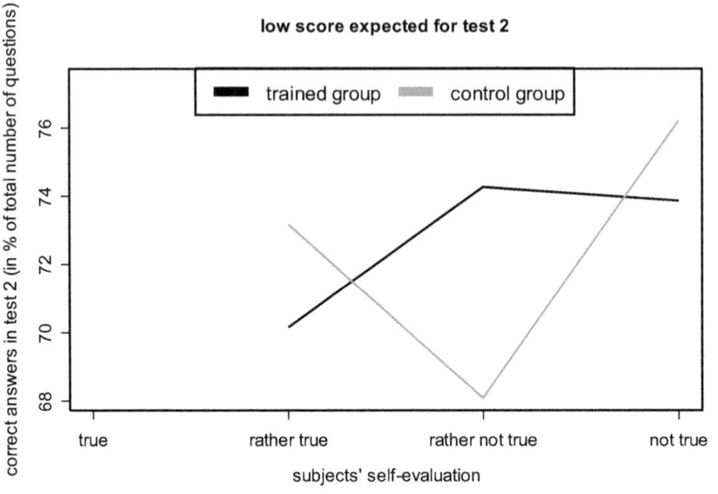

figure A.3-106: responses to the statement of a low score expected for test 2 juxtaposed with the percentage of questions answered correctly in test 2

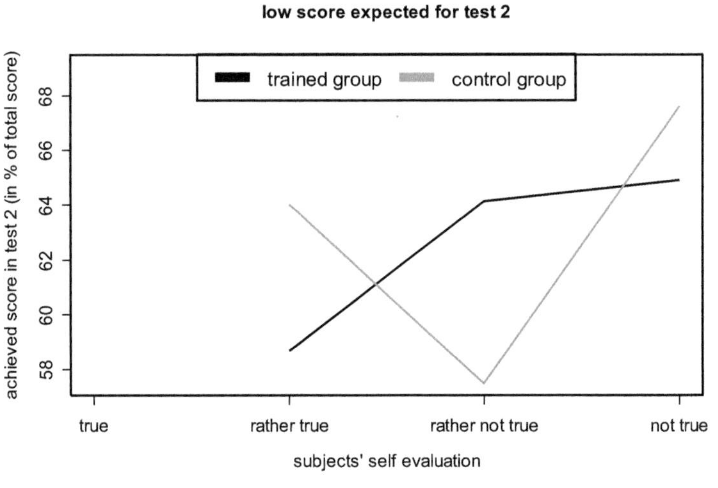

figure A.3-107: responses to the statement of a low score expected for test 2 juxtaposed with the percentage of the maximum score achieved in test 2

Appendix B Sound-Discrimination Test Questions and Answers

Appendix B.1 Pre-Intervention Test

question 1

acoustic input:	*Ostan tuon kirjan.* (I buy that book.)
question:	*Wie viele Wörter haben Sie gehört?* (How many words did you hear?)
answer options:	a) *1 Wort* (1 word) b) *2 Wörter* (2 words) c) *3 Wörter* (3 words) d) *4 Wörter* (4 words)
correct answer:	c
points for correct answer:	1

question 2

acoustic input:	*Isännän vieraat saapuivat myöhemmin.* (The guests of the landlord arrived later.)
question:	*Welches Wort haben Sie an der gekennzeichneten Stelle gehört?* _____ _____ __X__ _____ (Which word did you hear at the marked slot?)
answer options:	a) *isännän* (landlord's) b) *myöhemmin* (later) c) *saapuivat* (arrived – in 3rd person plural) d) *vieraat* (guests)
correct answer:	c
points for correct answer:	5

question 3

acoustic input:	*rumaa* (ugly – in partitive[232])
question:	*Welches dieser Wörter haben Sie gehört?* (Which of the following words did you hear?)
answer options:	a) *ruma* (ugly) b) *rumaa* (ugly – in partitive singular) c) *ruuma* (cargo compartment) d) *ruumaa* (cargo compartment – in partitive singular)
correct answer:	b
points for correct answer:	7

232 As previously explained in chapter 4, *partitiivi* (partitive) is one of the fifteen cases in Finnish. It is used to express an indefinite quantity of something and occurs with nouns as well as with their describing adjectives as in the context described above. It is comparable to the partitive use of *de* in French, such as in *Je bois du lait.* (I drink milk.).

question 4

acoustic input: *Voitteko odottaa huoneessa.* (Please wait in the room. [in polite form of address])

question: *An welcher Stelle haben Sie das Wort „huoneessa"* *gehört?* (In what position did you hear the word "in the room"]?)

answer options:
a) *an erster Stelle* (in first position)
b) *an zweiter Stelle* (in second position)
c) *an dritter Stelle* (in third position)

correct answer: c

points for correct answer: 2

question 5

question: *Welches der gehörten Beispiele ist das Wort „ilmanmuutoksessa"?* (Which of the heard examples is the word "in the weather change"?)

acoustic answer options:
a) *ilmeenmuutoksessa* (in the change of expression)
b) *ilmanmuutoksessa* (in the weather change)
c) *ilmanmuutoksia* (weather changes – in partitive)
d) *ilmanmuutoksesta* (out of the weather change)
e) *ilmeenmuutoksesta* (out of the change of expression)

correct answer: b

points for correct answer: 6

question 6

acoustic input: *Isot tytöt ovat täällä.* (The big girls are here.)

question: *In welcher Reihenfolge haben Sie diese Wörter gehört?* (In which order did you hear these words?)

answer options:
a) *isot* (big – in plural)
b) *ovat* (are)
c) *täällä* (here)
d) *tytöt* (girls)

correct answer: a, d, b, c

points for correct answer: 4

question 7

acoustic input: *Runsaskätiset merkkihenkilöt rahoittavat taidetta.* (The generous celebrities fund art.)

question: *Welches Wort im folgenden Satz weicht vom gehörten Satz ab? „Avokätiset merkkihenkilöt rahoittavat taidetta."* (Which word of the following sentence differs from the heard sentence? "The prodigal celebrities funded art.")

answer options:
a) *avokätiset* (prodigal – in plural)
b) *merkkihenkilöt* (celebrities)
c) *rahoittavat* (fund – in 3rd person plural)
d) *taidetta* (art – in partitive)

correct answer: a

points for correct answer: 6

question 8

question: *Welcher der gehörten Sätze ist der Satz „Hän on vanha."?* (Which of the heard sentences is the sentence "He is old."?)

acoustic answer options:
a) *Hän oli vanha.* (He was old.)
b) *Hän on kiva.* (He is nice.)
c) *Hän on vanha.* (He is old.)

correct answer: c

points for correct answer: 1

question 9

acoustic input: *Isoäiti merkitsi lapsenlapsen syntymäpäivän kalenteriin.* (The grandmother marked the grandchild's birthday in the calendar.)

question: *An welcher Stelle haben Sie das Wort „merkitsi" gehört?* (In what position did you hear the word "marked"?)

answer options:
a) an erster Stelle (in first position)
b) an zweiter Stelle (in second position)
c) an dritter Stelle (in third position)
d) an vierter Stelle (in fourth position)
e) an fünfter Stelle (in fifth position)

correct answer: b

points for correct answer: 8

question 10

acoustic input: *Tieteenharjoittajan ennakkoluulot vahvistuivat.* (The scientists' prejudice was reinforced.)

question: Welches Wort im folgenden Satz weicht vom gehörten Satz ab? *„Luonnonparantajan ennakkoluulot vahvistuivat."* (Which word of the following sentence differs from the heard sentence? "The naturopath's preconceptions were reinforced.")

answer options:
a) *luonnonparantajan* (the naturopath's)
b) *ennakkoluulot* (prejudice)
c) *vahvistuivat* (reinforced – in 3rd person plural)

correct answer: a

points for correct answer: 3

question 11

acoustic input: *turva* (protection)

question: *Welches dieser Wörter haben Sie gehört?* (Which of the following words did you hear?)

answer options:
a) *turha* (in vain)
b) *turma* (accident)
c) *turpa* (mouth – for animals or in rude language)
d) *turta* (numb)
e) *turva* (protection)

correct answer: e

points for correct answer: 4

question 12

acoustic input: *Aurinko paistoi yhdeksän tuntia.* (The sun was shining for nine hours.)

question: *In welcher Reihenfolge haben Sie diese Wörter gehört?* (In which order did you hear these words?)

answer options:
a) *aurinko* (the sun)
b) *paistoi* (shone – in 3rd person singular)
c) *tuntia* (hours – in partitive singular)
d) *yhdeksän* (nine)

correct answer: a, b, d, c

points for correct answer: 5

question 13

acoustic input: *Kaupungitkin tarjoavat mielenkiintoisia luonnonläheisiä opiskeluympäristöjä.* (The cities offer interesting nature-orientated study environments as well.)

question: *Wie viele Wörter haben Sie gehört?* (How many words did you hear?)

answer options:
a) *3 Wörter* (3 words)
b) *4 Wörter* (4 words)
c) *5 Wörter* (5 words)
d) *6 Wörter* (6 words)
e) *7 Wörter* (7 words)

correct answer: c

points for correct answer: 9

question 14

question: *Welches der gehörten Beispiele ist das Wort „puuhun"?* (Which of the heard examples is the word "into the tree"?)

acoustic answer options:
a) *puuhunsa* (into his tree)
b) *puuhunhan* (into the tree indeed)
c) *puuhunkin* (into the tree, too)
d) *puu* (tree)
e) *puuhun* (into the tree)

correct answer: e

points for correct answer: 1

question 15

acoustic input: *Mieheni kalastaa lomalla.* (My husband goes fishing on holidays.)

question: *Welches Wort haben Sie an der gekennzeichneten Stelle gehört?*

_____ __X__ _____

(Which word did you hear at the marked slot?)

answer options:
a) *kalastaa* (goes fishing)
b) *lomalla* (on holidays)
c) *mieheni* (my husband)

correct answer: a

points for correct answer: 2

question 16

question:	*Welcher der gehörten Sätze ist der Satz „Missä kirjasi nyt on?"?* (Which of the heard sentences is the sentence "Where is your book now?"?)
acoustic answer options:	a) *Missä kirjani nyt on?* (Where is my book now?) b) *Missä kirjasi nyt on?* (Where is your book now?) c) *Missä kirjansa nyt on?* (Where is his/her book now?)
correct answer:	b
points for correct answer:	4

question 17

acoustic input:	*Liikkeenhoitajat myöntyivät vastentahtoisesti pienehköihin palkankorotuksiin työaikojensa pidennyttyä.* (The managers reluctantly agreed on smaller pay rises after the extension of their working hours.)
question:	*Welches Wort haben Sie an der gekennzeichneten Stelle gehört?* ____ ____ ____ ____ _X_ ____ ____ (Which word did you hear at the marked slot?)
answer options:	a) *liikkeenhoitajat* (the managers) b) *myöntyivät* (agreed – in 3rd person plural) c) *palkankorotuksiin* (pay rise – in illative[233]) d) *pidennyttyä* (extended – past participle passive) e) *pienehköihin* (smaller) f) *työaikojensa* (their working hours) g) *vastentahtoisesti* (reluctantly)
correct answer:	c
points for correct answer:	9

question 18

acoustic input:	*viikonloppu* (weekend)
question:	*Welches dieser Wörter haben Sie gehört?* (Which of the following words did you hear?)
answer options:	a) *viikonloppu* (weekend) b) *viikonloppuja* (weekends – in partitive) c) *viikonlopulle* (towards the weekend) d) *viikonlopulla* (on the weekend) e) *viikonloppuna* (at the weekend)
correct answer:	a
points for correct answer:	2

question 19

question:	*Welches der gehörten Beispiele ist das Wort „sokka"?* (Which of the heard examples is the word "split pin"]?)
acoustic answer options:	a) *sokki* (shock) b) *sakka* (deposit) c) *sokko* (blindman's buff) d) *sokka* (split pin)

233 Illative is the inner local case in Finnish expressing a movement into an inward direction.

	e) *sika* (pig)
correct answer:	d
points for correct answer:	4

question 20

acoustic input:	*Talonomistajat neuvottelevat viikonloppuna remonttitöistä.* (The house owners discuss about renovation works at the weekend.)
question:	*In welcher Reihenfolge haben Sie diese Wörter gehört?* (In which order did you hear these words?)
answer options:	a) *neuvottelevat* (discuss – in 3rd person plural) b) *remonttitöistä* (out of renovation works) c) *talonomistajat* (house owners) d) *viikonloppuna* (at the weekend)
correct answer:	c, a, d, b
points for correct answer:	6

question 21

acoustic input:	*Kohtasimme lomalla Ranskassa yhdeksän vuotta sitten.* (We spent our holidays in France nine years ago.)
question:	*Wie viele Wörter haben Sie gehört?* (How many words did you hear?)
answer options:	a) *3 Wörter* (3 words) b) *4 Wörter* (4 words) c) *5 Wörter* (5 words) d) *6 Wörter* (6 words) e) *7 Wörter* (7 words)
correct answer:	d
points for correct answer:	8

question 22

acoustic input:	*Minä tunnen sinut.* (I know you.)
question:	*An welcher Stelle haben Sie das Wort „sinut" gehört?* (In what position did you hear the word "you"?)
answer options:	a) *an erster Stelle* (in first position) b) *an zweiter Stelle* (in second position) c) *an dritter Stelle* (in third position)
correct answer:	c
points for correct answer:	1

question 23

question:	Welcher der gehörten Sätze ist der Satz „*Huomenna kirjoitan äidille.*"? (Which of the heard sentences is the sentence "Tomorrow, I'll write Mother."?)
acoustic answer options:	a) *Tänään kirjoitan äidille.* (Today, I'll write Mother.) b) *Huomenna kirjoitan ruotsiksi.* (Tomorrow, I'll write in Swedish.) c) *Huomenna kirjoitan äidille.* (Tomorrow, I'll write Mother.)
correct answer:	c
points for correct answer:	2

question 24

acoustic input:	*Koira on pöydän alla.* (The dog is under the table.)
question:	*Welches Wort im folgenden Satz weicht vom gehörten Satz ab? „Koira oli pöydän alla."* (Which word of the following sentence differs from the heard sentence? "The dog was under the table.")
answer options:	a) *koira* (dog) b) *oli* (was) c) *pöydän* (the table's) d) *alla* (under)
correct answer:	b
points for correct answer:	4

question 25

acoustic input:	*Postinkantajat pysyttelivät lyhytaikaisesti sisätiloissa ukkossateen alettua.* (The post men temporarily stayed in confined spaces after the beginning of a thunder storm.)
question:	*An welcher Stelle haben Sie das Wort „sisätiloissa" gehört?* (In what position did you hear the word "confined spaces"?)
answer options:	a) *an erster Stelle* (in first position) b) *an zweiter Stelle* (in second position) c) *an dritter Stelle* (in third position) d) *an vierter Stelle* (in fourth position) e) *an fünfter Stelle* (in fifth position) f) *an sechster Stelle* (in sixth position)
correct answer:	d
points for correct answer:	9

question 26

acoustic input:	*maassa* (in the country)
question:	*Welches dieser Wörter haben Sie gehört?* (Which of the following words did you hear?)
answer options:	a) *maa* (country) b) *maassa* (in the country) c) *maassakin* (in the country, too) d) *maassako* (in the country?) e) *maassani* (in my country)
correct answer:	b
points for correct answer:	1

question 27

acoustic input:	*Koululaiset syövät ranskalaisia perunoita.* (The pupils eat potato chips.)
question:	*Welches Wort in diesem Satz weicht vom gehörten Satz ab? „Koululaiset söivät ranskalaisia perunoita."* (Which word of the following sentence differs from the heard sentence? "The pupils ate potato chips.")
answer options:	a) *koululaiset* (pupils) b) *söivät* (ate – in 3rd person plural)

c) *ranskalaisia* (French – in partitive plural)
d) *perunoita* (potatoes – in partitive)

correct answer: b
points for correct answer: 5

question 28
acoustic input: *Maahanmuuttajat ymmärsivät kysymykset.* (The immigrants understood the questions.)
question: *Welches Wort haben Sie an der gekennzeichneten Stelle gehört?*
_____ __X__ _____
(Which word did you hear at the marked slot?)
answer options:
a) *kysymykset* (questions)
b) *maahanmuuttajat* (immigrants)
c) *ymmärsivät* (understood – in 3rd person plural)

correct answer: c
points for correct answer: 3

question 29
question: *Welches der gehörten Beispiele ist das Wort „siika"?* (Which of the heard examples is the word "whitefish"?)
acoustic answer options:
a) *sika* (pig)
b) *sikaa* (pig – in partitive)
c) *siika* (whitefish)
d) *siikaa* (whitefish – in partitive)

correct answer: c
points for correct answer: 7

question 30
acoustic input: *Ymmärtääkö vaimonne venäjää?* (Does your wife understand Russian?)
question: *In welcher Reihenfolge haben Sie diese Wörter gehört?* (In which order did you hear these words?)
answer options:
a) *vaimonne* (your wife – in polite form of address)
b) *venäjää* (Russian)
c) *ymmärtääkö* (understand – in 3rd person singular with interrogative suffix)

correct answer: c, a, b
points for correct answer: 2

question 31
acoustic input: *Lastentarhalapset tuijottavat antiikkista siipirataslaivaa.* (The kindergarten children stare at an antique paddle steamer.)
question: *Wie viele Wörter haben Sie gehört?* (How many words did you hear?)
answer options:
a) *3 Wörter* (3 words)
b) *4 Wörter* (4 words)
c) *5 Wörter* (5 words)
d) *6 Wörter* (6 words)
e) *7 Wörter* (7 words)

correct answer: b
points for correct answer: 6

question 32

question: *Welcher der gehörten Sätze ist der Satz „Etsimme koiraani kahdeksan tuntia."?* (Which of the heard sentences is the sentence "We were looking for my dog for eight hours."?)

acoustic answer options:
a) *Etsimme koiraani yhdeksän tuntia.* (We were looking for my dog for nine hours.)
b) *Etsimme koiraani kahdeksan tuntia.* (We were looking for my dog for eight hours.)
c) *Etsimme koiraasi kahdeksan tuntia.* (We were looking for your dog for eight hours.)

correct answer: b
points for correct answer: 5

question 33

acoustic input: *Olen siellä kaksi päivää.* (I am there for two days.)

question: *An welcher Stelle haben Sie das Wort „kaksi" gehört?* (In what position did you hear the word "two"?)

answer options:
a) *an erster Stelle* (in first position)
b) *an zweiter Stelle* (in second position)
c) *an dritter Stelle* (in third position)
d) an vierter Stelle (in fourth position)

correct answer: c
points for correct answer: 4

question 34

acoustic input: *Luonnonsuojelijat varoittivat mahdollisista muuttuvista luonnonilmiöistä.* (The conservationists warned of possibly changing nature phenomena.)

question: *In welcher Reihenfolge haben Sie diese Wörter gehört?* (In which order did you hear these words?)

answer options:
a) *luonnonilmiöistä* (nature phenomena – in elative[234] plural)
b) *luonnonsuojelijat* (conservationists)
c) *mahdollisista* (possible – in elative plural)
d) *muuttuvista* (changing – in elative plural)
e) *varoittivat* (warned – in 3rd person plural)

correct answer: b, e, c, d, a
points for correct answer: 9

question 35

acoustic input: *Menetkö ravintolaan syömään?* (Do you go to the restaurant for lunch/dinner?[235])

---

234 Elative is one of the six local cases in Finnish. It is employed to express an outward directed movement. In the case of this sentence, it is required by the preceding verb varoittaa (to warn).

235 *Syömään* literally translates as "for eating".

question: *Welches Wort im folgenden Satz weicht vom gehörten Satz ab? „Menetkö ruokalaan syömään?"* (Which word of the following sentence differs from the heard sentence? "Do you go to the cafeteria for lunch?")
answer options: a) *menetkö* (do you go?)
b) *ruokalaan* (into the cafeteria)
c) *syömään* (to eat – in illative singular of the 3rd infinitive[236])
correct answer: b
points for correct answer: 2

question 36
question: *Welches der gehörten Beispiele ist das Wort „syntymäpäivä"?* (Which of the heard examples is the word "birthday"?)
acoustic answer options: a) *syntymäpäiväni* (my birthday)
b) *syntymäpäiviä* (birthdays – in partitive)
c) *syntymäpäivälle* (birthday – in allative[237])
d) *syntymäpäiväsi* (your birthday)
e) *syntymäpäivä* (birthday)
correct answer: e
points for correct answer: 3

question 37
acoustic input: *Oli kiva nähdä sinut taas.* (It was nice to see you again.)
question: *Wie viele Wörter haben Sie gehört?* (How many words did you hear?)
answer options: a) *3 Wörter* (3 words)
b) *4 Wörter* (4 words)
c) *5 Wörter* (5 words)
d) *6 Wörter* (6 words)
e) 7 Wörter (7 words)
correct answer: c
points for correct answer: 7

question 38
acoustic input: *Viime viikolla virkamies soitteli virastolle kymmenen kertaa.* (Last week, the magistrate called the authorities ten times.)
question: *Welches Wort haben Sie an der gekennzeichneten Stelle gehört?*
____ ____ __X__ ____ ____ ____ ___
(Which word did you hear at the marked slot?)
answer options: a) *kertaa* (times – in partitive singular)
b) *kymmenen* (ten)
c) *soitteli* (called – in 3rd person singular)

236 The 3rd infinitive in Finnish is employed in verb-nominalisation contexts.
237 Allative is one of the six local cases in Finnish. It is applied for the expression of a movement towards something.

d) *viikolla* (week – in adessive[238])
e) *viime* (last)
f) *virastolle* (authorities – in allative)
g) *virkamies* (magistrate)

correct answer: g
points for correct answer: 8

question 39

acoustic input: *kirjeeni* (my letter)
question: *Welches dieser Wörter haben Sie gehört?* (Which of the following words did you hear?)
answer options:
a) *kirjani* (my book)
b) *kirjasi* (your book)
c) *kirjeeni* (my letter)
d) *kirjeensä* (his/her letter)
e) *kirjeesi* (your letter)

correct answer: c
points for correct answer: 5

question 40

question: *Welcher der gehörten Sätze ist der Satz „Osoitelapulleni kirjoitettiin virheellinen osoitetieto."?* (Which of the heard sentences is the sentence "Wrong address details were written on my address label."?)
acoustic answer options:
a) *Osoitelipulleni kirjoitettiin virheellinen osoitetieto.* (Wrong address details were written on my address ticket.)
b) *Osoitelapulleni kirjoitettiin virheellinen osoitetieto.* (Wrong address details were written on my address label.)
c) *Osoitelapullesi kirjoitettiin virheellinen osoitetieto.* (Wrong address details were written on your address label.)

correct answer: b
points for correct answer: 6

question 41

acoustic input: *Eilen menin kauppaan ja ostin uuden kirjan.* (Yesterday, I went to the shop and bought a new book.)
question: *In welcher Reihenfolge haben Sie diese Wörter gehört?* (In which order did you hear these words?)
answer options:
a) *eilen* (yesterday)
b) *ja* (and)
c) *kauppaan* (into the shop)
d) *kirjan* (the book – in genitive accusative[239])
e) *menin* (went – in 1st person singular)

238 Adessive is one of the six local cases in Finnish. It is applied to express the position on top of something. In the present case, it is used in a temporal context expressing a time span.

239 The genitive accusative in Finnish is a formal genitive taking the place and function of a direct object.

	f) *ostin* (bought – in 1st person singular)
	g) *uuden* (new – in genitive)
correct answer:	a, e, c, b, f, g, d
points for correct answer:	7

question 42

question:	*Welches der gehörten Beispiele ist das Wort „rajalla"?* (Which of the heard examples is the word "on the border"?)
acoustic answer options:	a) *rajalta* (from the border)
	b) *rahalla* (with money)
	c) *rajalle* (towards the border)
	d) *rajalla* (on the border)
	e) *rahalta* (from the money)
correct answer:	d
points for correct answer:	5

question 43

acoustic input:	*puhelinkoppi* (telephone booth)
question:	*Welches dieser Wörter haben Sie gehört?* (Which of the following words did you hear?)
answer options:	a) *puhelinkopille* (towards the telephone booth)
	b) *puhelinkoppi* (telephone booth)
	c) *puhelinkopissa* (in the telephone booth)
	d) *puhelinkopilla* (at the telephone booth)
	e) *puhelinkopista* (out of the telephone booth)
correct answer:	b
points for correct answer:	3

question 44

acoustic input:	*Tullitarkastajat tiedottavat osoitteenmuutoksen rekisteritoimistolle.* (The customs officers inform the registration office of the address change.)
question:	*An welcher Stelle haben Sie das Wort „osoitteenmuutoksen" gehört?* (In what position did you hear the word "the address change's"?)
answer options:	a) *an erster Stelle* (in first position)
	b) *an zweiter Stelle* (in second position)
	c) *an dritter Stelle* (in third position)
	e) an vierter Stelle (in fourth position)
correct answer:	c
points for correct answer:	6

question 45

acoustic input:	*Se on uusi talo.* (It is a new house.)
question:	*Wie viele Wörter haben Sie gehört?* (How many words did you hear?)
answer options:	a) *3 Wörter* (3 words)
	b) *4 Wörter* (4 words)
	c) *5 Wörter* (5 words)

d) *6 Wörter* (6 words)
correct answer: b
points for correct answer: 4

question 46
acoustic input: *Olen kirkon takana.* (I am behind the church.)
question: *Welches Wort im folgenden Satz weicht vom gehörten Satz ab? „Olen kirkon edessä."* (Which word of the following sentence differs from the heard sentence? "I am in front of the church.")
answer options:
a) *olen* (I am)
b) *kirkon* (the church's)
c) *edessä* (in the front)
correct answer: c
points for correct answer: 1

question 47
question: *Welcher der gehörten Sätze ist der Satz „Ylipäälliköt pysäköivät kulkuneuvot."?* (Which of the heard sentences is the sentence "The commanders-in-chief parked the vehicles."?)
acoustic answer options:
a) *Ylipäälliköt pysäköivät kulkuneuvot.* (The commanders-in-chief parked the vehicles.)
b) *Ylipäälliköt pysäköivät panssariajoneuvot.* (The commanders-in-chief parked the tanks.)
c) *Autonkuljettajat pysäköivät kulkuneuvot.* (The drivers parked the vehicles.)
correct answer: a
points for correct answer: 3

question 48
acoustic input: *Sinä et ole kiva.* (You are not nice.)
question: *Welches Wort haben Sie an der gekennzeichneten Stelle gehört?*
_____ _____ __X__ _____
(Which word did you hear at the marked slot?)
answer options:
a) *et* (not – in 3rd person singular)
b) *kiva* (nice)
c) *ole* (be – negated form, indicative, present, active)
d) *sinä* (you)
correct answer: c
points for correct answer: 4

question 49
acoustic input: *Yöpyykö ystäväsi siellä?* (Does your friend stay there overnight?)
question: *Wie viele Wörter haben Sie gehört?* (How many words did you hear?)
answer options:
a) *2 Wörter* (2 words)
b) *3 Wörter* (3 words)

	c) *4 Wörter* (4 words)
	d) *5 Wörter* (5 words)
	e) *6 Wörter* (6 words)
correct answer:	b
points for correct answer:	2

question 50

acoustic input:	*Ruokaosaston toimihenkilöt ihmettelivät.* (The staff of the food section was wondering.)
question:	*In welcher Reihenfolge haben Sie diese Wörter gehört?* (In which order did you hear these words?)
answer options:	a) *ihmettelivät* (wondered – in 3rd person plural)
	b) *ruokaosaston* (the food section's)
	c) *toimihenkilöt* (staff)
correct answer:	b, c, a
points for correct answer:	3

question 51

acoustic input:	*Toivon, että hän ei ole täällä.* (I hope that he/she is not here.)
question:	*An welcher Stelle haben Sie das Wort „hän" gehört?* (In what position did you hear the word "he/she"?)
answer options:	a) *an erster Stelle* (in first position)
	b) *an zweiter Stelle* (in second position)
	c) *an dritter Stelle* (in third position)
	d) an vierter Stelle (in fourth position)
	e) *an fünfter Stelle* (in fifth position)
	f) *an sechster Stelle* (in sixth position)
correct answer:	c
points for correct answer:	7

question 52

acoustic input:	*voimistelunopettajaksi* (to a physical education teacher)
question:	*Welches dieser Wörter haben Sie gehört?* (Which of the following words did you hear?)
answer options:	a) *voimistelunopettajasi* (your physical education teacher)
	b) *voimistelunopettajani* (my physical education teacher)
	c) *voimistelunopettajaksi* (to a physical education teacher)
	d) *voimistelunopettajansa* (his/her physical education teacher)
	e) *voimistelunopettajasta* (from the physical education teacher)
correct answer:	c
points for correct answer:	6

question 53

acoustic input:	*Äiti ei tule tänään, koska hän on sairas.* (Mother is not coming today because she is ill.)
question:	*Welches Wort haben Sie an der gekennzeichneten Stelle gehört?*
	____ ____ __X__ ____ ____ ____ ____ ____

	(Which word did you hear at the marked slot?)
answer options:	a) *äiti* (mother) b) *ei* (not – in 3rd person singular) c) *hän* (she) d) *koska* (because) e) *on* (is) f) *sairas* (ill) g) *tänään* (today) h) *tule* (come)
correct answer:	h
points for correct answer:	7

question 54

acoustic input:	*Hän on kotona.* (He/she is at home.)
question:	*In welcher Reihenfolge haben Sie diese Wörter gehört?* (In which order did you hear these words?)
answer options:	a) *hän* (he/she) b) *kotona* (at home) c) *on* (is)
correct answer:	a, c, b
points for correct answer:	1

question 55

question:	*Welches der gehörten Beispiele ist das Wort „vieras"?* (Which of the heard examples is the word "guest"?)
acoustic answer options:	a) *vierastaa* (to be shy with strangers) b) *vierastan* (I am shy with strangers.) c) *vierasta* (guest – in partitive) d) *vierastat* (You are shy with strangers.) e) *vieras* (guest)
correct answer:	e
points for correct answer:	5

question 56

acoustic input:	*Näkövammaiset oppisopimusoppilaat unohtavat kotitehtävät.* (The visually impaired trainees forget their homework.)
question:	*Welches Wort haben Sie an der gekennzeichneten Stelle gehört?* _____ __X__ _____ _____ (Which word did you hear at the marked slot?)
answer options:	a) *kotitehtävät* (homework) b) *näkövammaiset* (visually impaired) c) *oppisopimusoppilaat* (trainees) d) *unohtavat* (forget – in 3rd person plural)
correct answer:	c
points for correct answer:	6

question 57

acoustic input:	*Kirjallisuusarvostelijat rentoutuvat kuntoutuslaitoksessa.* (The literature critics relax in a convalescent home.)

question:	*Wie viele Wörter haben Sie gehört?* (How many words did you hear?)
answer options:	a) *3 Wörter* (3 words) b) *4 Wörter* (4 words) c) *5 Wörter* (5 words) d) *6 Wörter* (6 words) e) 7 Wörter (7 words)
correct answer:	b
points for correct answer:	3

question 58

acoustic input:	*Onko teillä kylpyamme mökillä?* (Do you have a bath tub in your summer house?)
question:	*An welcher Stelle haben Sie das Wort „teillä" gehört?* (In what position did you hear the word "you"?)
answer options:	a) *an erster Stelle* (in first position) b) *an zweiter Stelle* (in second position) c) *an dritter Stelle* (in third position) d) *an vierter Stelle* (in fourth position)
correct answer:	b
points for correct answer:	5

question 59

acoustic input:	*Panen kirjan laukkuun.* (I put the book into the bag.)
question:	*Welches Wort haben Sie an der gekennzeichneten Stelle gehört?* ____ ____ __X__ (Which word did you hear at the marked slot?)
answer options:	a) *kirjan* (book – in genitive accusative) b) *laukkuun* (into the bag) c) *panen* (I put)
correct answer:	b
points for correct answer:	1

question 60

acoustic input:	*Taiteenharrastajat matkustivat purjelentokoneella.* (The amateur artists travelled by sailplane.)
question:	*An welcher Stelle haben Sie das Wort „purjelentokoneella" gehört?* (In what position did you hear the word "by sailplane"?)
answer options:	a) *an erster Stelle* (in first position) b) *an zweiter Stelle* (in second position) c) *an dritter Stelle* (in third position)
correct answer:	c
points for correct answer:	3

question 61

acoustic input:	*Huomenna olemme kotona syömässä.* (Tomorrow we are at home for lunch/dinner. [literally: for eating])
question:	*Wie viele Wörter haben Sie gehört?* (How many words did you hear?)

answer options: a) *3 Wörter* (3 words)
b) *4 Wörter* (4 words)
c) *5 Wörter* (5 words)
d) *6 Wörter* (6 words)
e) 7 Wörter (7 words)
correct answer: b
points for correct answer: 5

question 62
acoustic input: *Utelias vieras maisteli montaa ruokaa.* (The curious guest tried many foods.)
question: *In welcher Reihenfolge haben Sie diese Wörter gehört?* (In which order did you hear these words?)
answer options: a) *maisteli* (tried – in 3rd person singular)
b) *montaa* (many – in partitive)
c) *ruokaa* (food – in partitive)
d) *utelias* (curious)
e) *vieras* (guest)
correct answer: d, e, a, b, c
points for correct answer: 8

Appendix B.2 Post-Intervention Test

question 1

acoustic input: *Ostan tämän kukan.* (I buy this flower.)
question: *Wie viele Wörter haben Sie gehört?* (How many words did you hear?)
answer options:
a) *1 Wort* (1 word)
b) *2 Wörter* (2 words)
c) *3 Wörter* (3 words)
d) *4 Wörter* (4 words)
correct answer: c
points for correct answer: 1

question 2

acoustic input: *Vieraat saapuivat myöhemmin laivalla.* (The guests arrived by boat later.)
question: *Welches Wort haben Sie an der gekennzeichneten Stelle gehört?*
_____ _____ __X__ _____
(Which word did you hear at the marked slot?)
answer options:
a) *laivalla* (on the boat)
b) *myöhemmin* (later)
c) *saapuivat* (arrived – in 3rd person plural)
d) *vieraat* (guests)
correct answer: b
points for correct answer: 5

question 3

acoustic input: *pulla* [pulla[240]]
question: *Welches dieser Wörter haben Sie gehört?* (Which of the following words did you hear?)
answer options:
a) *pula* (lack)
b) *pulaa* (lack – in partitive)
c) *pulla* (pulla)
d) *pullaa* (pulla – in partitive)
e) puulla (on the tree)
correct answer: c
points for correct answer: 7

question 4

acoustic input: *Voitteko nukkua sängyssä.* (Please sleep in the bed. [in polite form of address])
question: *An welcher Stelle haben Sie das Wort „nukkua" gehört?* (In what position did you hear the word "in the bed"?)
answer options:
a) *an erster Stelle* (in first position)
b) *an zweiter Stelle* (in second position)
c) *an dritter Stelle* (in third position)

240 traditional Finnish yeast pastry

correct answer: b
points for correct answer: 2

question 5
question: *Welches der gehörten Beispiele ist das Wort „verinäytteestä"?* (Which of the heard examples is the word "from the blood sample"?)
acoustic answer options:
a) *verinäytteessä* (in the blood sample)
b) *verinäytteestä* (out of the blood sample)
c) *värinäytteessä* (in the colour sample)
d) *värinäytteestä* (out of the colour sample)
e) *verinäytteeseen* (into the blood sample)
correct answer: b
points for correct answer: 6

question 6
acoustic input: *Iso poika meni pois.* (The big boy went away.)
question: *In welcher Reihenfolge haben Sie diese Wörter gehört?* (In which order did you hear these words?)
answer options:
a) *iso* (big)
b) *meni* (went – in 3rd person singular)
c) *poika* (boy)
d) *pois* (away)
correct answer: a, c, b, d
points for correct answer: 4

question 7
acoustic input: *Oopperalaulajat esiintyivät viikonloppuisin ahkerasti.* (The opera singers performed diligently on the weekends.)
question: *Welches Wort im folgenden Satz weicht vom gehörten Satz ab? „Oopperalaulajat esiintyvät viikonloppuisin ahkerasti."* (Which word of the following sentence differs from the heard sentence? "The opera singers perform diligently on the weekends.")
answer options:
a) *ooperalaulajat* (the opera singers)
b) *esiintyvät* (perfom – in 3rd person plural)
c) *viikonloppuisin* (the weekends')
d) *ahkerasti* (diligently)
correct answer: b
points for correct answer: 6

question 8
question: *Welcher der gehörten Sätze ist der Satz „Hän on kiva."?* (Which of the heard sentences is the sentence "He is nice.")
acoustic answer options:
a) *Hän on vanha.* (He is old.)
b) *Hän on kiva.* (He is nice.)
c) *Hän oli kiva.* (He was nice.)
correct answer: b
points for correct answer: 1

question 9
acoustic input: *Opettaja merkitsi koululaisen syntymäpäivän kalenteriin.* (The teacher marked the pupil's birthday in the calendar.)
question: *An welcher Stelle haben Sie das Wort „koululaisen"* *gehört?* (In what position did you hear the word "pupil"?)
answer options: a) an erster Stelle (in first position)
b) an zweiter Stelle (in second position)
c) an dritter Stelle (in third position)
d) an vierter Stelle (in fourth position)
e) an fünfter Stelle (in fifth position)
correct answer: c
points for correct answer: 8

question 10
acoustic input: *Tähtitieteilijän olettamukset vahvistuivat.* (The astronomers' hypotheses proved true.)
question: Welches Wort im folgenden Satz weicht vom gehörten Satz ab? *„Luonnontieteilijän olettamukset vahvistuivat."* (Which word of the following sentence differs from the heard sentence? "The natural scientist's hypotheses proved true")
answer options: a) *luonnontieteilijän* (the natural scientists')
b) *olettamukset* (hypotheses)
c) *vahvistuivat* (proved true)
correct answer: a
points for correct answer: 3

question 11
acoustic input: *mummo* (granny)
question: *Welches dieser Wörter haben Sie gehört?* (Which of the following words did you hear?)
answer options: a) *mummi* (grandma)
b) *mummin* (grandma's)
c) *mummo* (granny)
d) *mummu* (granny)
e) *muna* (egg)
correct answer: c
points for correct answer: 4

question 12
acoustic input: *Lapsenlapsi kuunteli isoäidin kertomusta.* (The grandchild listened to the grandmother's story.)
question: *In welcher Reihenfolge haben Sie diese Wörter gehört?* (In which order did you hear these words?)
answer options: a) *isoäidin* (the grandmother's)
b) *kertomusta* (story – in partitive)
c) *kuunteli* (listened – in 3rd person singular)
d) *lapsenlapsi* (grandchild)
correct answer: d, c, a, b
points for correct answer: 5

question 13

acoustic input: *Maanomistajien vaatimukset otettiinkin eduskunnassa käsittelylistalle.* (The land owners' claims were added to the negotiation list.)

question: *Wie viele Wörter haben Sie gehört?* (How many words did you hear?)

answer options:
a) *3 Wörter* (3 words)
b) *4 Wörter* (4 words)
c) *5 Wörter* (5 words)
d) *6 Wörter* (6 words)
e) *7 Wörter* (7 words)

correct answer: c

points for correct answer: 9

question 14

question: *Welches der gehörten Beispiele ist das Wort „jäällä"?* (Which of the heard examples is the word "on the ice"]?)

acoustic answer options:
a) *jäällä* (on the ice)
b) *jää* (ice)
c) *jäälläkö* (on the ice?)
d) *jäälläkään* (neither on the ice)
e) *jäällämme* (on our ice)

correct answer: a

points for correct answer: 1

question 15

acoustic input: *Vaimoni kirjoittaa runoja.* (My wife writes poems.)

question: *Welches Wort haben Sie an der gekennzeichneten Stelle gehört?*

_____ __X__ _____

(Which word did you hear at the marked slot?)

answer options:
a) *kirjoittaa* (writes)
b) *runoja* (poems – in partitive)
c) *vaimoni* (my wife)

correct answer: a

points for correct answer: 2

question 16

question: *Welcher der gehörten Sätze ist der Satz „Missä veljesi on ollut?"?* (Which of the heard sentences is the sentence "Where has your brother been?"?)

acoustic answer options:
a) *Missä veljeni on ollut?* (Where has my brother been?)
b) *Missä veljesi on ollut?* (Where has your brother been?)
c) *Missä veljemme on ollut?* (Where has our brother been?)

correct answer: b

points for correct answer: 4

question 17

acoustic input:	*Jääkiekkojoukkueen huoltajatkin erehtyivät turnauksen päivämäärästä.* (Also the attendants of the icehockey team were mistaken in the date of the tournament.)
question:	*Welches Wort haben Sie an der gekennzeichneten Stelle gehört?* ____ ____ _X_ ____ ____ (Which word did you hear at the marked slot?)
answer options:	a) *erehtyivät* (were mistaken – in 3rd person plural) b) *huoltajatkin* (also the attendants) c) *jääkiekkojoukkueen* (the icehockey team's) d) *päivämäärästä* (in the date) e) *turnauksen* (the tournament's)
correct answer:	a
points for correct answer:	9

question 18

acoustic input:	*joululoma* (Christmas holidays)
question:	*Welches dieser Wörter haben Sie gehört?* (Which of the following words did you hear?)
answer options:	a) *joululoma* (Christmas holidays) b) *joululomalla* (on Christmas holidays) c) *joululomalle* (towards the Christmas holidays) d) *joululomalta* (from the Christmas holidays) e) *joululomani* (my Christmas holidays)
correct answer:	a
points for correct answer:	2

question 19

question:	*Welches der gehörten Beispiele ist das Wort „solut"?* (Which of the heard examples is the word "cells"?)
acoustic answer options:	a) *solmu* (knot) b) *solu* (cell) c) *solut* (cells) d) *solun* (the cell's) e) *solmun* (the knot's)
correct answer:	c
points for correct answer:	4

question 20

acoustic input:	*Puutarhurit istuttavat lauantaisin ruusupensaita.* (The gardeners planted rosebushes on Saturdays.)
question:	*In welcher Reihenfolge haben Sie diese Wörter gehört?* (In which order did you hear these words?)
answer options:	a) *istuttavat* (dibbled – in 3rd person plural) b) *lauantaisin* (on Saturdays) c) *puutarhurit* (gardeners) d) *ruusupensaita* (rosebushes – in partitive)
correct answer:	c, a, b, d
points for correct answer:	6

question 21
acoustic input: *Naapurimme kohtasivat lomalla Ruotsissa kymmenen vuotta sitten.* (Our neighbours met on holidays in Sweden ten years ago.)
question: *Wie viele Wörter haben Sie gehört?* (How many words did you hear?)
answer options: a) *3 Wörter* (3 words)
b) *4 Wörter* (4 words)
c) *5 Wörter* (5 words)
d) *6 Wörter* (6 words)
e) *7 Wörter* (7 words)
correct answer: e
points for correct answer: 8

question 22
acoustic input: *Hän muistaa minut.* (He remembers me.)
question: *An welcher Stelle haben Sie das Wort „minut" gehört?* (In what position did you hear the word "me"?)
answer options: a) *an erster Stelle* (in first position)
b) *an zweiter Stelle* (in second position)
c) *an dritter Stelle* (in third position)
correct answer: c
points for correct answer: 1

question 23
question: Welcher der gehörten Sätze ist der Satz „*Tänään odotan sinua.*"? (Which of the heard sentences is the sentence "I'm waiting for you today."?)
acoustic answer options: a) *Tänään odotan kissaa.* (I'm waiting for the cat today.)
b) *Huomenna odotan sinua.* (I'll wait for you tomorrow.)
c) *Tänään odotan sinua.* (I'm waiting for you today.)
correct answer: c
points for correct answer: 2

question 24
acoustic input: *Kissa on pöydän päällä.* (The cat is on the table.)
question: *Welches Wort im folgenden Satz weicht vom gehörten Satz ab? „Koira on pöydän päällä."* (Which word of the following sentence differs from the heard sentence? "The dog is on the table.")
answer options: a) *koira* (dog)
b) *on* (is)
c) *pöydän* (the table's)
d) *päällä* (on the top)
correct answer: a
points for correct answer: 4

question 25
acoustic input: *Kuntalaiset järjestivät jokavuotiset perinteiset urheilukilpailut.* (The inhabitants of the district organised the annual traditional sports competitions.)

question: *An welcher Stelle haben Sie das Wort „perinteiset" gehört?* (In what position did you hear the word "traditional"?)
answer options:
a) *an erster Stelle* (in first position)
b) *an zweiter Stelle* (in second position)
c) *an dritter Stelle* (in third position)
d) *an vierter Stelle* (in fourth position)
e) *an fünfter Stelle* (in fifth position)
correct answer: d
points for correct answer: 9

question 26
acoustic input: *kuussa* (in the moon)
question: *Welches dieser Wörter haben Sie gehört?* (Which of the following words did you hear?)
answer options:
a) *kuu* (moon)
b) *kuussa* (in the moon)
c) *kuussakaan* (neither in the moon)
d) *kuussakin* (in the moon, too)
e) *kuussako* (in the moon?)
correct answer: b
points for correct answer: 1

question 27
acoustic input: *Urheilijat syövät keitettyjä perunoita.* (The sportsmen eat cooked potatoes.)
question: *Welches Wort in diesem Satz weicht vom gehörten Satz ab? „Urheilijat söivät keitettyjä perunoita."* (Which word of the following sentence differs from the heard sentence? "The sportsmen ate cooked potatoes.")
answer options:
a) *urheilijat* (the sportsmen)
b) *söivät* (ate – in 3rd person plural)
c) *keitettyjä* (cooked – in partitive plural)
d) *perunoita* (potatoes – in partitive)
correct answer: b
points for correct answer: 5

question 28
acoustic input: *Saamelaiset harjoittavat poronkasvatusta.* (The Lapps breed reindeer.)
question: *Welches Wort haben Sie an der gekennzeichneten Stelle gehört?*
_____ __X__ _____
(Which word did you hear at the marked slot?)
answer options:
a) *harjoittavat* (practice – in 3rd person plural)
b) *poronkasvatusta* (reindeer breeding – in partitive)
c) *saamelaiset* (Lapps)
correct answer: a
points for correct answer: 3

question 29
question: *Welches der gehörten Beispiele ist das Wort „mutaa"?* (Which of the heard examples is the word "mud"?)
acoustic answer options: a) *mutta* (but)
b) *mutaa* (mud – in partitive)
c) *muta* (mud)
d) *muuta* (other – in partitive)
correct answer: b
points for correct answer: 7

question 30
acoustic input: *Ymmärtääkö veljesi ruotsia?* (Does your brother understand Swedish?)
question: *In welcher Reihenfolge haben Sie diese Wörter gehört?* (In which order did you hear these words?)
answer options: a) *ruotsia* (Swedish)
b) *veljesi* (your brother)
c) *ymmärtääkö* (understand – in 3rd person singular with interrogative suffix)
correct answer: c, b, a
points for correct answer: 2

question 31
acoustic input: *Ruotsikoululaiset vierailivat paikallisella lentokentällä.* (The Swedish pupils visited the local airport.)
question: *Wie viele Wörter haben Sie gehört?* (How many words did you hear?)
answer options: a) *3 Wörter* (3 words)
b) *4 Wörter* (4 words)
c) *5 Wörter* (5 words)
d) *6 Wörter* (6 words)
e) *7 Wörter* (7 words)
correct answer: b
points for correct answer: 6

question 32
question: *Welcher der gehörten Sätze ist der Satz „Etsimme kissaasi kahdeksan tuntia."?* (Which of the heard sentences is the sentence "We were looking for your cat for eight hours."?)
acoustic answer options: a) *Etsimme kissaasi yhdeksän tuntia.* (We were looking for your cat for nine hours.)
b) *Etsimme kissaani kahdeksan tuntia.* (We were looking for my dog for eight hours.)
c) *Etsimme kissaasi kahdeksan tuntia.* (We were looking for your dog for eight hours.)
correct answer: c
points for correct answer: 5

question 33

acoustic input: *Juhla kestää kolme päivää.* (The celebration lasts three days.)

question: *An welcher Stelle haben Sie das Wort „päivää" gehört?* (In what position did you hear the word "days"?)

answer options:
a) *an erster Stelle* (in first position)
b) *an zweiter Stelle* (in second position)
c) *an dritter Stelle* (in third position)
d) an vierter Stelle (in fourth position)

correct answer: d

points for correct answer: 4

question 34

acoustic input: *Sairaanhoitajat luokiteltiin pienipalkkaisiin hoitoalan työntekijöihin.* (Nurses were categorised into nursing professions with low wages.)

question: *In welcher Reihenfolge haben Sie diese Wörter gehört?* (In which order did you hear these words?)

answer options:
a) *hoitoalan* (of the nursing sector)
b) *luokiteltiin* (were categorised)
c) *pienipalkkaisiin* (into low wages)
d) *sairaanhoitajat* (nurses)
e) *työntekijöihin* (staff)

correct answer: d, b, c, a, e

points for correct answer: 9

question 35

acoustic input: *Menemme siellä uimaan.* (We go there for swimming.)

question: *Welches Wort im folgenden Satz weicht vom gehörten Satz ab? „Menemme siellä lukemaan."* (Which word of the following sentence differs from the heard sentence? "We go there for reading.")

answer options:
a) *menemme* (we go)
b) *siellä* (there)
c) *lukemaan* (to read – in illative singular of the 3rd infinitive)

correct answer: c

points for correct answer: 2

question 36

question: *Welches der gehörten Beispiele ist das Wort „sienikeitto"?* (Which of the heard examples is the word "mushroom soup"?)

acoustic answer options:
a) *sienikeittoa* (mushroom soup – in partitive)
b) *sienikeitossa* (in the mushroom soup)
c) *sienikeitosta* (out of the mushroom soup)
d) *sienikeittoja* (mushroom soups – in partitive)
e) *sienikeitto* (mushroom soup)

correct answer: e

points for correct answer: 3

question 37

acoustic input: *Oli hauska nähdä hänet taas.* (It was a pleasure to see him/her again.)

question: *Wie viele Wörter haben Sie gehört?* (How many words did you hear?)

answer options:
a) *3 Wörter* (3 words)
b) *4 Wörter* (4 words)
c) *5 Wörter* (5 words)
d) *6 Wörter* (6 words)
e) 7 Wörter (7 words)

correct answer: c

points for correct answer: 7

question 38

acoustic input: *Viime vuonna matruusi soitteli äidille satakaksi kertaa.* (Last year, the sailor called his mother a hundred and two times.)

question: *Welches Wort haben Sie an der gekennzeichneten Stelle gehört?*

____ ____ ____ ____ _X_ _____ ___

(Which word did you hear at the marked slot?)

answer options:
a) *äidille* (to the mother)
b) *kertaa* (times – in partitive singular)
c) *matruusi* (sailor)
d) *satakaksi* (a hundred and two)
e) *soitteli* (called – in 3rd person singular)
f) *viime* (last)
g) *vuonna* (year – in essive[241])

correct answer: a

points for correct answer: 8

question 39

acoustic input: *lappuni* (my slip of paper)

question: *Welches dieser Wörter haben Sie gehört?* (Which of the following words did you hear?)

answer options:
a) *lappuni* (my slip of paper)
b) *lappunsa* (his/her slip of paper)
c) *lappusi* (your slip of paper)
d) *lippuni* (my ticket)
e) *lippusi* (your ticket)

correct answer: a

points for correct answer: 5

question 40

question: *Welcher der gehörten Sätze ist der Satz „Kahvikannusi kuuluivatkin erikoiseen astiastoon."?* (Which of the heard sentences is the sentence "Your coffeepot does belong to a special tablewear."?)

---

241 Essive is one of the fifteen cases in Finnish. It is applied in temporal contexts.

acoustic answer options: a) *Kahvikannuni kuuluivatkin erikoiseen astiastoon.* (My coffeepot does belong to a special tablewear.)
b) *Kahvipannuni kuuluivatkin erikoiseen astiastoon.* (My coffee kettle does belong to a special tablewear.)
c) *Kahvikannusi kuuluivatkin erikoiseen astiastoon.* (Your coffeepot does belong to a special tablewear.)
correct answer: c
points for correct answer: 6

question 41
acoustic input: *Nainen meni kauppaan ja osti kauniin kukan.* (The woman went to the shop and bought a pretty flower.)
question: *In welcher Reihenfolge haben Sie diese Wörter gehört?* (In which order did you hear these words?)
answer options: a) *ja* (and)
b) *kauniin* (pretty – in genitive)
c) *kauppaan* (into the shop)
d) *kukan* (flower – in genitive accusative)
e) *meni* (went – in 3rd person singular)
f) *nainen* (woman)
g) *osti* (bought – in 3rd person singular)
correct answer: f, e, c, a, g, b, d
points for correct answer: 7

question 42
question: *Welches der gehörten Beispiele ist das Wort „majalta"?* (Which of the heard examples is the word "from the shed"?)
acoustic answer options: a) *majalta* (from the shed)
b) *mahalla* (on the stomach)
c) *majalle* (towards the shed)
d) *majalla* (at the shed)
e) *mahalta* (from the stomach)
correct answer: a
points for correct answer: 5

question 43
acoustic input: *postilaatikko* (postbox)
question: *Welches dieser Wörter haben Sie gehört?* (Which of the following words did you hear?)
answer options: a) *postilaatikko* (postbox)
b) *postilaatikolla* (at the postbox)
c) *postilaatikolta* (from the postbox)
d) *postilaatikossa* (in the postbox)
e) *postilaatikosta* (out of the postbox)
correct answer: a
points for correct answer: 3

question 44

acoustic input: *Esitelmöijät kummastelivat epäpäteviä kysymyksiä.* (The lecturers were surprised about the unqualified questions.)

question: *An welcher Stelle haben Sie das Wort „epäpäteviä"* *gehört?* (In what position did you hear the word "unqualified"?)

answer options:
a) *an erster Stelle* (in first position)
b) *an zweiter Stelle* (in second position)
c) *an dritter Stelle* (in third position)
e) an vierter Stelle (in fourth position)

correct answer: c

points for correct answer: 6

question 45

acoustic input: *Mies osti uuden veneen.* (The man bought a new boat.)

question: *Wie viele Wörter haben Sie gehört?* (How many words did you hear?)

answer options:
a) *3 Wörter* (3 words)
b) *4 Wörter* (4 words)
c) *5 Wörter* (5 words)
d) *6 Wörter* (6 words)

correct answer: b

points for correct answer: 4

question 46

acoustic input: *Olen talon takana.* (I am behind the house.)

question: *Welches Wort im folgenden Satz weicht vom gehörten Satz ab? „Olen talon edessä."* (Which word of the following sentence differs from the heard sentence? "I am in front of the church.")

answer options:
a) *olen* (I am)
b) *talon* (the house's)
c) *edessä* (in the front)

correct answer: c

points for correct answer: 1

question 47

question: *Welcher der gehörten Sätze ist der Satz „Palopäällikkö valmistautuu harjoituksiin?"?* (Which of the heard sentences is the sentence "The fire brigade's officer-in-charge gets ready for the practice."?)

acoustic answer options:
a) *Palopäällikkö valmistautuu harjoituksiin?* (The fire brigade's officer-in-charge gets ready for the practice.)
b) *Palopäällikkö valmistautuu sammuttamaan.* (The fire brigade's officer-in-charge gets ready for extinguishing the fire.)
c) *Merimies valmistautuu harjoituksiin.* (The sailor gets ready for the practice.)

correct answer: a

points for correct answer: 3

question 48
acoustic input: *Tyttö oli oikein kiva.* (The girl was very nice.)
question: *Welches Wort haben Sie an der gekennzeichneten Stelle gehört?*
_____ __X__ _____ _____
(Which word did you hear at the marked slot?)
answer options:
a) *kiva* (nice)
b) *oikein* (very)
c) *oli* (was – in 3rd person singular)
d) *tyttö* (the girl)
correct answer: c
points for correct answer: 4

question 49
acoustic input: *Asuvatko lääkärit kotona?* (Do the doctors live at home?)
question: *Wie viele Wörter haben Sie gehört?* (How many words did you hear?)
answer options:
a) *2 Wörter* (2 words)
b) *3 Wörter* (3 words)
c) *4 Wörter* (4 words)
d) *5 Wörter* (5 words)
e) *6 Wörter* (6 words)
correct answer: b
points for correct answer: 2

question 50
acoustic input: *Korkeakoulun opiskelijat tupakoivat.* (The university students smoke.)
question: *In welcher Reihenfolge haben Sie diese Wörter gehört?* (In which order did you hear these words?)
answer options:
a) *korkeakoulun* (the university's)
b) *opiskelijat* (students)
c) *tupakoivat* (smoke – in 3rd person plural)
correct answer: b, c, a
points for correct answer: 3

question 51
acoustic input: *Luulen, että hän ei ole täällä.* (I think that he/she is not here.)
question: *An welcher Stelle haben Sie das Wort „ole" gehört?* (In what position did you hear the word "be"?)
answer options:
a) *an erster Stelle* (in first position)
b) *an zweiter Stelle* (in second position)
c) *an dritter Stelle* (in third position)
d) an vierter Stelle (in fourth position)
e) *an fünfter Stelle* (in fifth position)
f) *an sechster Stelle* (in sixth position)
correct answer: e
points for correct answer: 7

question 52

acoustic input: *uskonnonopettajansa* (his/her religious education teacher)
question: *Welches dieser Wörter haben Sie gehört?* (Which of the following words did you hear?)
answer options:
a) *uskonnonopettajaksi* (to a religious education teacher)
b) *uskonnonopettajani* (my religious education teacher)
c) *uskonnonopettajansa* (his/her religious education teacher)
d) *uskonnonopettajasi* (your religious education teacher)
e) *uskonnonopettajasta* (from the religious education teacher)
correct answer: c
points for correct answer: 6

question 53

acoustic input: *Lapsi ei tahdo tulla kotiin, koska hän leikkii.* (The child does not want to come home because he/she is playing.)
question: *Welches Wort haben Sie an der gekennzeichneten Stelle gehört?*
____ ____ _X_ ____ ____ ____ ____ ____
(Which word did you hear at the marked slot?)
answer options:
a) *ei* (not – in 3rd person singular)
b) *hän* (he/she)
c) *koska* (because)
d) *kotiin* (home – in illative)
e) *lapsi* (child)
f) *leikkii* (plays)
g) *tahdo* (want)
h) *tulla* (come)
correct answer: g
points for correct answer: 7

question 54

acoustic input: *Hän on sairas.* (He/she is ill.)
question: *In welcher Reihenfolge haben Sie diese Wörter gehört?* (In which order did you hear these words?)
answer options:
a) *hän* (he/she)
b) *on* (is)
c) *sairas* (ill)
correct answer: a, b, c
points for correct answer: 1

question 55

question: *Welches der gehörten Beispiele ist das Wort „sokeri"?* (Which of the heard examples is the word "sugar"?)
acoustic answer options:
a) *sokeria* (sugar – in partitive)
b) *sokerissa* (in the sugar)
c) *sokeri* (sugar)
d) *sokerista* (out of the sugar)
e) *sokerinsa* (his/her sugar)

correct answer: c
points for correct answer: 5

question 56

acoustic input: *Hyväntuuliset kirkkovaltuutetut lörpöttelivät kirkastussunnuntaina.* (The good-humoured parish representatives chatted on Whitsunday.)

question: *Welches Wort haben Sie an der gekennzeichneten Stelle gehört?*

_____ __X__ _____ _____

(Which word did you hear at the marked slot?)

answer options:
a) *hyväntuuliset* (good-humoured)
b) *lörpöttelivät* (catted – in 3rd person plural)
c) *kirkastussunnuntaina* (on Whitsunday)
d) *kirkkovaltuutetut* (parish representatives)

correct answer: d
points for correct answer: 6

question 57

acoustic input: *Yhteiskuntatieteilijät rentoutuvat lähivirkistysaluella.* (The social scientists relaxed in the local recreation area.)

question: *Wie viele Wörter haben Sie gehört?* (How many words did you hear?)

answer options:
a) *3 Wörter* (3 words)
b) *4 Wörter* (4 words)
c) *5 Wörter* (5 words)
d) *6 Wörter* (6 words)
e) 7 Wörter (7 words)

correct answer: a
points for correct answer: 3

question 58

acoustic input: *Tykkäättekö uimisesta järvissä kesällä?* (Do you like swimming in the lakes in summer?)

question: *An welcher Stelle haben Sie das Wort „uimisesta" gehört?* (In what position did you hear the word "swimming"?)

answer options:
a) *an erster Stelle* (in first position)
b) *an zweiter Stelle* (in second position)
c) *an dritter Stelle* (in third position)
d) *an vierter Stelle* (in fourth position)

correct answer: b
points for correct answer: 5

question 59

acoustic input: *Panen kellon laukkuun.* (I put the clock into the bag.)

question: *Welches Wort haben Sie an der gekennzeichneten Stelle gehört?*

_____ __X__ _____

(Which word did you hear at the marked slot?)

answer options:
a) *kellon* (clock – in genitive accusative)
b) *laukkuun* (into the bag)

	c) *panen* (put – in 1st person singular)
correct answer:	b
points for correct answer:	1

question 60

acoustic input:	*Uutistenlukijat matkustivat maanalaisella.* (The newsreaders travelled by underground.)
question:	*An welcher Stelle haben Sie das Wort „matkustivat"* *gehört?* (In what position did you hear the word "travelled"?)
answer options:	a) *an erster Stelle* (in first position)
	b) *an zweiter Stelle* (in second position)
	c) *an dritter Stelle* (in third position)
correct answer:	b
points for correct answer:	3

question 61

acoustic input:	*Huomenna olemme takaisin kotona.* (Tomorrow, we are back home.)
question:	*Wie viele Wörter haben Sie gehört?* (How many words did you hear?)
answer options:	a) *3 Wörter* (3 words)
	b) *4 Wörter* (4 words)
	c) *5 Wörter* (5 words)
	d) *6 Wörter* (6 words)
	e) 7 Wörter (7 words)
correct answer:	b
points for correct answer:	5

question 62

acoustic input:	*Pormestarin siskontytär opiskelee ruotsia Tukholmassa.* (The mayor's niece studies Swedish in Stockholm.)
question:	*In welcher Reihenfolge haben Sie diese Wörter gehört?* (In which order did you hear these words?)
answer options:	a) *opiskelee* (studies)
	b) *pormestarin* (the mayor's)
	c) *ruotsia* (Swedish)
	d) *siskontytär* (neice)
	e) *Tukholmassa* (in Stockholm)
correct answer:	b, d, a, c, e
points for correct answer:	8

Appendix C Questionnaires

Appendix C.1 Pre-Examination Survey on the Subjects' Prior Language Learning and Musical Habits

A: questions on previous foreign-language experience:

A.1 foreign languages learned at school
Did you learn one or more foreign language(s) at school? ☐ yes ☐ no → Please proceed with item **A.2.**

A.1.1 your first foreign language at school
What was the first foreign language you learned at school?

For how many years did you learn this language? year(s)

Are you still using this language on a daily basis? ☐ yes ☐ no

Did you continue learning this language in a course after finishing school (also at a later point of time)? ☐ yes ☐ no → Please proceed with item **A.1.2.**

How long did you attend this course? year(s)

Are you still learning this language? ☐ yes → Please proceed with item **A.1.2.** ☐ no

How many years have passed since the end of this course? year(s)

A.1.2 your second foreign language at school
Did you learn a second foreign language at school? ☐ yes ☐ no → Please proceed with item **A.2.**

What was the second foreign language you learned at school?

For how many years did you learn this language? year(s)

Are you still using this language on a daily basis? ☐ yes ☐ no

Did you continue learning this language in a course after finishing school (also at a later point of time)? ☐ yes ☐ no → Please proceed with item **A.1.3.**

How long did you attend this course? year(s)

Are you still learning this language? ☐ yes → Please proceed with item **A.1.3.** ☐ no

How many years have passed since the end of this course? year(s)

A.1.3 your third foreign language at school
Did you learn a third foreign language at school? ☐ yes ☐ no → Please proceed with item **A.2.**

What was the third foreign language you learned at school?

For how many years did you learn this language? year(s)

Are you still using this language on a daily basis? ☐ yes ☐ no

Did you continue learning this language in a course after finishing school (also at a later point of time)? ☐ yes ☐ no → Please proceed with item **A.1.4.**

How long did you attend this course? year(s)

Are you still learning this language? ☐ yes → Please proceed with item **A.1.4.** ☐ no

How many years have passed since the end of this course? year(s)

A.1.4 your fourth foreign language at school

Did you learn a fourth foreign language at school? ☐ yes ☐ no → Please proceed with item **A.2.**

What was the fourth foreign language you learned at school?

For how many years did you learn this language? year(s)

Are you still using this language on a daily basis? ☐ yes ☐ no

Did you continue learning this language in a course after finishing school (also at a later point of time)? ☐ yes ☐ no → Please proceed with item **A.2.**

How long did you attend this course? year(s)

Are you still learning this language? ☐ yes → Please proceed with item **A.2.** ☐ no

How many years have passed since the end of this course? year(s)

A.2 foreign languages learned in extracurricular courses in your own country

Did you learn any further foreign language in an extracurricular course in your own country? ☐ yes ☐ no → Please proceed with item **A.3.**

A.2.1 your first extracurricular foreign language in your own country

Which language did you take a course in?

How long did you learn this language? year(s)

Are you still using this language on a daily basis? ☐ yes ☐ no

Are you still learning this language? ☐ yes → Please proceed with item **A.2.2.** ☐ no

How many years have passed since the end of this course? year(s)

A.2.2 your second extracurricular foreign language in your own country

Did you learn a further foreign language in an extracurricular course in your own country? ☐ yes ☐ no → Please proceed with item **A.3.**

Which language did you take a course in?

How long did you learn this language? year(s)

Are you still using this language on a daily basis? ☐ yes ☐ no

Are you still learning this language? ☐ yes → Please proceed with item **A.2.3.** ☐ no

How many years have passed since the end of this course? year(s)

A.2.3 your third extracurricular foreign language in your own country
Did you learn a further foreign language in an extracurricular course in your own country? ☐ yes ☐ no → Please proceed with item **A.3.**

Which language did you take a course in?

How long did you learn this language? year(s)

Are you still using this langue on a daily basis? ☐ yes ☐ no

Are you still learning this language? Please proceed with item **A.3.** ← ☐ yes ☐ no

How many years have passed since the end of this course? year(s)

A.3 foreign-language courses abroad
Did you take part in one more language course(s) aboroad? ☐ yes ☐ no → Please proceed with item **A.4.**

A.3.1 language courses abroad in one of the above stated languages

A.3.1.1 your first course abroad in an already learned language
Did you extend your knowledge in one of the above stated languages in a language course abroad? ☐ yes ☐ no → Please proceed with item **A.3.2.**

Which of the above stated foreign languages does this apply for?

How long did you stay abroad? weeks

How long did your course abroad take? weeks

A.3.1.2 your second course abroad in an already learned language
Did you extend your knowledge in a further of the above stated languages in a language course abroad? ☐ yes ☐ no → Please proceed with item **A.3.2.**

Which of the above stated foreign languages does this apply for?

How long did you stay abroad? weeks

How long did your course abroad take? weeks

A.3.2 language courses abroad in new foreign languages

A.3.2.1 your first course abroad in a new foreign language
Did you learn a new foreign language in a course abroad? ☐ yes ☐ no → Please proceed with item **A.4.**

Which new language did you learn abroad?

How long did you stay abroad? weeks

How long did your course abroad take? weeks

Are you still using this language on a daily basis? ☐ yes ☐ no

A.3.2.2 your second course abroad in a new foreign language
Did you learn a further new foreign language in a course abroad? ☐ yes ☐ no → Please proceed with item **A.4.**

Which further language did you learn abroad?

How long did you stay abroad? weeks

How long did your course abroad take? weeks

Are you still using this language on a daily basis? ☐ yes ☐ no

A.4 further foreign languages learned in other contexts

A.4.1 your first further language
Did you learn a further foreign language in a different context? ☐ yes ☐ no → Please proceed with item **B.**

Which further language did you learn?

In which context did you learn this language?

How long did you learn this language? year(s)

Are you still using this language on a daily basis? ☐ yes ☐ no

Are you still learning this language? Please proceed with item **A.4.2.** ← ☐ yes ☐ no

How many years have passed since you stopped learning this language? year(s)

A.4.2 your second further language
Did you learn a further language in a different context? ☐ yes ☐ no → Please proceed with item **B.**

Which further language did you learn?

In which context did you learn this language?

How long did you learn this language? year(s)

Are you still using this language on a daily basis? ☐ yes ☐ no

Are you still learning this language? Please proceed with item **B.** ← ☐ yes ☐ no

How many years have passed since you stopped learning this language? year(s)

B: questions on daily exposure to music

B.1 your listening habits

B.1.1 type of music most listened to
B.1.1a
Which type of music do you listen to most frequently?

How much time **per day** do you spend on actively listening to this music? hour(s)

How much time **per day** do you keep this music passively playing in the background? hour(s)

Do you sometimes actively take part in the music by singing or drumming along? ☐ yes ☐ no → Please proceed with item **B.1.1b.**

Do you sometimes sing along to the music?	☐ yes ☐ no →	Please proceed **at** * below.
Do you sing the main melody?	☐ yes ☐ no	
Do you sing a different voice from the music?	☐ yes ☐ no	
Do you invent a new voice matching the music?	☐ yes ☐ no	
* Do you sometimes drum or tap along to the music with your hands, fingers or feet?	☐ yes ☐ no →	Please proceed with item **B.1.1b**.
Do you drum or tap the general beat of the music?	☐ yes ☐ no	
Do you drum or tap a different rhythm occurring in the music?	☐ yes ☐ no	
Do you drum or tap a self-invented rhythm matching the music?	☐ yes ☐ no	

B.1.2 other types of music you listen to
Which other types of music do you sometimes listen to?

How much time **per week** do you spend on actively listening to these types of music?	hour(s)	
How much time **per week** do you keep this music passively playing in the background?	hour(s)	
Do you sometimes actively take part in the music by singing or drumming along?	☐ yes ☐ no →	Please proceed with item **B.2**.
Do you sometimes sing along to the music?	☐ yes ☐ no →	Please proceed **at** * below.
Do you sing the main melody?	☐ yes ☐ no	
Do you sing a different voice from the music?	☐ yes ☐ no	
Do you invent a new voice matching the music?	☐ yes ☐ no	
* Do you sometimes drum or tap along to the music with your hands, fingers or feet?	☐ yes ☐ no →	Please proceed with item **B.2**.
Do you drum or tap the general beat of the music?	☐ yes ☐ no	
Do you drum or tap a different rhythm occurring in the music?	☐ yes ☐ no	
Do you drum or tap a self-invented rhythm matching the music?	☐ yes ☐ no	

B.2 your musical environment
In which situations and contexts do you see yourself confronted with music in everyday life?

How do you react to this kind of music?	annoyed ☐ ☐ ☐ ☐ ☐ ☐ interested	
Do you have the same taste in music as your friends?	☐ absolutely → ☐ mostly ☐ rather not ☐ not at all	Please proceed with item **B.3**.
In the company of your friends, do you sometimes listen to types of music you normally wouldn't listen to?	☐ yes ☐ no →	Please proceed with item **B.3**.

How do you feel in those kind of situations? annoyed ☐ ☐ ☐ ☐ ☐ ☐ interested

B.3 your participation in musical life

B.3.1 live concerts
How often do you attend live concerts?

☐ never → Please proceed with item **B.3.2.**
☐ every 2 or 3 years
☐ once a year
☐ twice or thrice a year
☐ 4 to 5 times per year
☐ more often

Do you only attend concerts featuring a certain type of music? ☐ yes ☐ no

if yes: What is the type of music played at the concerts?

if no: Which types of music have you heard at live concerts so far?

B.3.2 festivals
How often do you attend music festivals?

☐ never → Please proceed with item **B.4.**
☐ less often than every 3rd year
☐ every 2 or 3 years
☐ once a year
☐ several times a year

Do you only attend festivals featuring a certain type of music? ☐ yes ☐ no

if yes: What is the type of music played at the festivals?

if no: Which types of music have you heard at festivals so far?

At the festivals, did you also listen to bands and artists playing other types of music? ☐ yes ☐ no → Please proceed with item **B.4.**

How did you feel at those occasions? annoyed ☐ ☐ ☐ ☐ ☐ ☐ interested

B.4 your self-classification

You have already found your music style and will stick to it.	true ☐ ☐ ☐ ☐ not true
You are always open for a new musical experience.	true ☐ ☐ ☐ ☐ not true
You just cannot get anything from some types of music.	true ☐ ☐ ☐ ☐ not true
You have dealt with many different types of music.	true ☐ ☐ ☐ ☐ not true
You cannot understand how somebody cannot like your favourite type of music.	true ☐ ☐ ☐ ☐ not true
You cannot understand that other people prefer other types of music.	true ☐ ☐ ☐ ☐ not true
You are still searching for your favourite type of music.	true ☐ ☐ ☐ ☐ not true
Your taste in music often changes.	true ☐ ☐ ☐ ☐ not true

Appendix C.2 Post-Examination Survey on the Subjects' Self-Evaluation

To me, the first sound-discrimination test was more difficult than the second.	true ☐ ☐ ☐ ☐ not true
To me, the second sound-discrimination test was more difficult than the first.	true ☐ ☐ ☐ ☐ not true
To me, both sound-discrimination tests were equally difficult.	true ☐ ☐ ☐ ☐ not true
I was able to get used to the sound of the new language right from the beginning of the first sound-discrimination test.	true ☐ ☐ ☐ ☐ not true
I was able to get used to the sound of the new language during the course of the two sound-discrimination tests.	true ☐ ☐ ☐ ☐ not true
I couldn't get used to the sound of the new language at all up to the end of the second sound-discrimination test.	true ☐ ☐ ☐ ☐ not true
During the second sound-discrimination test, I remembered sounds from the first.	true ☐ ☐ ☐ ☐ not true
The sounds from the first and the second sound-discrimination tests were completely different.	true ☐ ☐ ☐ ☐ not true
During the second sound-discrimination test, I remembered sound combinations from the first.	true ☐ ☐ ☐ ☐ not true
The sound combinations from the first and second sound-discrimination tests were completely different.	true ☐ ☐ ☐ ☐ not true
I had extreme difficulties with the first sound-discrimination test.	true ☐ ☐ ☐ ☐ not true
I had extreme difficulties with the second sound-discrimination test.	true ☐ ☐ ☐ ☐ not true
The first sound-discrimination test was extremely easy.	true ☐ ☐ ☐ ☐ not true
The second sound-discrimination test was extremely easy.	true ☐ ☐ ☐ ☐ not true
I think I answered the same number of questions correctly in both sound-discrimination tests.	true ☐ ☐ ☐ ☐ not true
I think I answered more questions correctly in the first sound-discrimination test than in the second.	true ☐ ☐ ☐ ☐ not true
I think I answered more questions correctly in the second sound-discrimination test than in the first.	true ☐ ☐ ☐ ☐ not true
I think I answered most questions correctly in the first sound-discrimination test.	true ☐ ☐ ☐ ☐ not true
I think I answered most questions correctly in the second sound-discrimination test.	true ☐ ☐ ☐ ☐ not true
I think I answered hardly any question correctly in the first sound-discrimination test.	true ☐ ☐ ☐ ☐ not true
I think I answered hardly any question correctly in the second sound-discrimination test.	true ☐ ☐ ☐ ☐ not true